DASH DIE_ _ _ _ _

COOKBOOK

A Detailed Guide to Lower Blood Pressure & Improve Your
Health

(Healthy Recipes for Naturally Weight Loss Solution)

Simon Smail

Published by Alex Howard

*Dash Diet for Beginners: A Detailed Guide to Lower Blood Pressure &
Improve Your Health (Healthy Recipes for Naturally Weight Loss Solution)*

ISBN 978-1-990169-61-8

Legal & Disclaimer

The information contained in this book is not designed to replace or take the place of any form of medicine or professional medical advice. The information in this book has been provided for educational and entertainment purposes only.

Table of contents

PART 1

INTRODUCTION

You are about to revolutionize your eating habits and it is going to be a life changing experience! If you have been suffering from hypertension (high blood pressure) or just want to start eating healthier and don't quite know what meals you need to introduce to your diet, worry no more. It's time to put the DASH in your diet and celebrate a healthy eating regime that it is highly recommended by medical and nutritional professionals and has been named the #1 leading diet by US News & World since 2011 for four consecutive years! DASH stands for **D**ietary **A**pproaches to **S**top **H**ypertension and has been intensively researched, coupled by scientific studies that show that it is the best diet towards hypertension and for anyone wanting to live a healthy lifestyle.

You have probably had the displeasure of experiencing conventional diet plans that restrict you from eating delicious and scrumptious meals. Why should you have to live through boring and flavorless food? Here is the fun part - this DASH Diet cookbook does not subscribe to that bland plan! Getting the right nutrition as well as visually admiring your artistic food is going to be the order of the day when it comes to the DASH Diet.

I have put together this handy and useful cookbook full of recipes compiled according to the endorsements of the DASH Diet. It contains many delicious recipes and mouth-watering meal plans that will make cooking fun and easy; whilst helping you to maintain good health. Foods such as processed can-foods, junk food, high fat items are highly discouraged. Whereas, home-cooked meals with fresh vegetables and fresh meat, and non-processed foods are highly welcomed and most certainly celebrated. This Dash Diet cookbook unlocks many recipes that encourage healing to take place in your body. Following these delectable, lip-smacking well thought-out healthy recipes will encourage an enjoyable lifestyle.

This cookbook contains a complete diet plan which includes tasty morning breakfast delights, healthy lunch meals, tasty snacks, savory soups, delicious salads, delectable dinner recipes, and of course desserts! Instructions and guidelines are simple and allow for a very easy, step by step meal preparation plan. Prepare yourself for a magical taste-bud adventure whilst your body starts regenerating itself and facilitating wellbeing at the same time. You know the drill, let's drop the bad eating habits, add a DASH of wonderment and let's get cooking!

BREAKFAST

Chicken Parmesan and Baked Quinoa

SERVINGS: **6**
PREP TIME: **20 min.**

TOTAL TIME: 1 hour

Ingredients

- 1 tablespoon olive oil
- 1 medium onion, diced
- 3 cloves garlic, minced
- 2 tablespoon balsamic vinegar
- 1 (15 oz.) can tomato sauce
- 1 (15 oz.) can diced tomatoes (no added salt)
- basil and oregano, to taste
- 1 cup quinoa
- 2 cups water or broth
- 1 lb. boneless, skinless chicken, cooked and cut into bite sized pieces
- 2/3 cup shredded part-skim mozzarella cheese, divided
- 2 tablespoon grated Parmesan or Romano cheese

Instructions

1. Preheat the oven to 375°F (190°C) and spray a 2 quart baking dish with cooking oil.
2. Heat a large skillet over medium heat and add oil. Stir in onion. Stir frequently for about 5-7 minutes, or until tender. Add garlic and cook until fragrant, about 30-60 seconds. Add the balsamic vinegar, mix and cook until it is nearly fully absorbed.
3. Add tomato sauce, diced tomatoes, basil, oregano, and pepper to taste. Bring to a low boil and then simmer while you make the rest of the meal.

4. Place quinoa in a mesh strainer. Rinse with cold water for 2 minutes.
5. In a small sauce pan, place quinoa and water or broth and bring to a boil (add a little salt if using water). Cover with a lid, reduce heat, and simmer until cooked, around 20-25 minutes.
6. Combine and mix the quinoa and chicken with the sauce in a large bowl.
7. Place mix in the baking dish and top with the mozzarella cheese and Parmesan.
8. Cover with foil and bake for about 15 minutes.
9. Remove foil and bake until cheese is bubbly and lightly browned, about 10 more minutes.

Raisins, Apples, and Cinnamon Granola

SERVINGS: **12**
PREP TIME: **15 min.**
TOTAL TIME: **1 hour**

Ingredients
- 1/4 cup slivered almonds
- 1/4 cup honey
- 1/4 cup unsweetened applesauce
- 1 tablespoon vanilla extract
- 1 tablespoon ground cinnamon
- 2 cups dry old-fashioned oatmeal
- 2 cups bran flakes
- 3/4 cup dried apple pieces
- 1/2 cup golden raisins

Instructions

1. Preheat the oven to 325°F (165°C). Lightly coat baking sheet with cooking spray.
2. Spread almonds on a baking sheet and bake. Stir occasionally for about 10 minutes, or until golden and fragrant. Transfer to a plate and cool. Raise temperature of the oven to 350°F (175°C).
3. In a small bowl, whisk honey, applesauce, vanilla and cinnamon together. Set aside.
4. Add oatmeal and bran flakes in a large bowl. Stir and mix well. Add honey mix and toss, being careful not to break the clumps apart.
5. Spread cereal mix evenly onto a baking sheet. Place in oven and stir occasionally. Bake until golden brown, about 30 minutes. Remove from oven and slightly cool.
6. Combine cereal mix, toasted almonds, apple pieces and raisins in a large bowl. Cool completely and store in an airtight container.

Mushroom Strata and Turkey Sausage Casserole

SERVINGS: **12**
PREP TIME: **15 min.**
TOTAL TIME: 1 hour + refrigeration

Ingredients

- 8 ounces wheat ciabatta bread, cut into 1-inch cubes
- 12 ounces turkey sausage
- 2 cups fat free milk
- 1-1/2 cup (4 ounces) reduced-fat shredded sharp cheddar cheese
- 3 large eggs
- 12 ounces egg substitute
- 1/2 cup chopped green onion
- 1 cup sliced mushrooms
- 1/2 teaspoon paprika
- Fresh ground pepper, to taste
- 2 tablespoons grated parmesan cheese

Instructions

1. Preheat oven to 400°F (200°C).
2. Arrange bread cubes on a baking sheet. Bake at 400°F (200°C) until toasted for about 8 minutes.
3. Heat a medium skillet over medium-high heat. Add sausage and cook 7 minutes or until browned. Stir to crumble.
4. In a large bowl combine milk, cheese, eggs, egg substitute, parmesan cheese, paprika, salt and pepper. Stir with a whisk.
5. Add bread, sausage, scallions and mushrooms. Toss well to coat bread. Spoon mix into a 13x9-inch baking dish. Cover and refrigerate for overnight or 8 hours.
6. Preheat oven to 350°F (175°C).

7. Uncover the casserole and bake for 50 minutes or until lightly browned.
8. Cut into 12 pieces and serve.

Blueberry-Raspberry Mint Gazpacho

SERVINGS: **4**

PREP TIME: **5 min.**

> **TOTAL TIME:** 15 min. + refrigeration

Ingredients

- 1 1/2 cups blueberries
- 1 1/2 cups raspberries
- 2 tablespoons sugar
- 1 tablespoon orange juice
- 1 teaspoon lemon juice
- 1 teaspoon lime juice
- 1 teaspoon lemon zest
- Fresh mint leaves, for garnish
- 4 scoops (1/4 cup each) fat-free Greek yogurt

Instructions

1. In a medium heatproof bowl, combine berries, sugar, orange, lemon and lime juice, and lemon zest.
2. Cover bowl with plastic wrap.
3. Place bowl over a large saucepan of simmering water and cook 10 minutes on low.
4. Set aside until it cools and refrigerate for about 4 hours.

5. Divide fruit and its liquid among 4 bowls. Garnish with fresh mint and top each with a 1/4 cup scoop of Greek yogurt.

Very Berry Muesli

SERVINGS: **4**

   PREP/TOTAL TIME: 10 min. + refrigeration

Ingredients

- 1 cup old-fashioned rolled oats (raw)
- 1 cup fruit yogurt
- 1/2 cup 1% milk
- Pinch of salt
- 1/2 cup dried fruit (raisins, apricots, dates)
- 1/2 cup chopped apple
- 1/2 cup frozen blueberries
- 1/4 cup chopped, toasted walnuts

Instructions

1. Mix oats, yogurt, milk and salt in medium bowl.
2. Cover and refrigerate overnight.
3. Add dried and fresh fruit. Mix gently.
4. Serve scoops of muesli in small dishes and sprinkle each serving with chopped nuts.
5. Refrigerate leftovers within 2-3 hours.

Avocado, Banana & Chocolate Pudding

SERVINGS: **6**

PREP TIME: **10 min.**
        TOTAL TIME: 1 hour 10 min

Ingredients

- 1 ripe avocado, peeled and pitted
- 4 very ripe bananas
- 1/4 cup unsweetened cocoa powder, plus more for garnish

Instructions

1. In a blender, blend avocados, bananas, and cocoa powder until smooth.
2. Pour into serving bowls and sprinkle additional cocoa powder on top.
3. Chill in refrigerator for at least 1 hour. Serve.

Banana-Oatmeal Pancake with Spiced Maple Syrup

SERVINGS: **6**
PREP TIME: **10 min.**
TOTAL TIME: **20 min.**

Ingredients

- 1/2 cup maple syrup
- 1/2 cinnamon stick
- 3 whole cloves
- 1/2 cup old-fashioned rolled oats
- 1 cup water
- 2 tablespoons firmly packed light brown sugar

- 2 tablespoons canola oil
- 1/2 cup whole-wheat/whole-meal flour
- 1/2 cup all-purpose plain flour
- 1 1/2 teaspoons baking powder
- 1/4 teaspoon baking soda
- 1/4 teaspoon salt
- 1/4 teaspoon ground cinnamon
- 1/2 cup 1 percent low-fat milk
- 1/4 cup fat-free plain yogurt
- 1 banana, peeled and mashed
- 1 egg, lightly beaten

Instructions

1. In a small saucepan, combine maple syrup, cinnamon stick and cloves. Place over medium heat and bring to a boil. Remove heat and let stand for 15 minutes. Remove the cinnamon stick and cloves with a slotted spoon and set syrup aside. Keep warm.
2. Combine oats and water in a large microwave-safe bowl. Microwave on high about 3 minutes or until oats are creamy and tender. Stir in the brown sugar and canola oil. Set aside to slightly cool.
3. Combine flours, baking powder, baking soda, salt and ground cinnamon in a bowl. Whisk to blend.
4. Add milk, yogurt and banana to oats and stir until well mixed. Beat in the egg. Add flour mix to the oat mix and stir just until moistened.
5. Heat a non-stick frying pan or griddle over medium heat. Spoon 1/4 cup pancake batter into the pan.

Cook until the top of pancake is covered with bubbles and the edges are slightly browned, about 2 minutes. Turn and cook until the bottom is well browned and the pancake is cooked through, about 1 to 2 more minutes. Repeat with the remaining pancake batter.

6. Place pancakes on warmed individual plates. Drizzle with the warm syrup and serve.

Breakfast Bread Pudding

SERVINGS: **4**
PREP TIME: **10 min.**
TOTAL TIME: **1 hour**

Ingredients

- 1 1/2 cup low fat or fat free milk
- 4 eggs
- 2 tablespoons brown sugar
- 1/2 teaspoon vanilla extract
- 1/2 teaspoon ground cinnamon
- 1/8 teaspoon salt
- 3 cups cubed whole wheat bread, about 4 slices
- 1/2 cup peeled and diced apple
- 1/4 cup raisins
- 2 teaspoons powdered sugar (optional)

Instructions

1. Preheat oven to 350°F (175°C).

2. Combine milk, eggs, brown sugar, vanilla, cinnamon and salt in a large bowl. Whisk until combined.
3. Add bread cubes, diced apple and raisins, and mix until all ingredients are combined and bread has soaked up most of the liquid.
4. Coat an 8-inch square baking dish with butter or non-stick spray.
5. Transfer bread mixture into the baking pan. Cover with foil.
6. Place bread pudding into the oven and bake for 40 minutes. Uncover and continue baking until golden brown, about 20 minutes more.
7. Let stand for 10 minutes before serving. Dust with powdered sugar, if desired.

Veggie Quiche Muffins

SERVINGS: **12**
PREP TIME: **10 min.**
TOTAL TIME: **45 min.**

Ingredients
- 3/4 cup low-fat cheddar cheese, shredded
- 1 cup green onion or onion, chopped
- 1 cup broccoli, chopped
- 1 cup tomatoes, diced
- 2 cups non-fat or 1% milk
- 4 eggs
- 1 cup baking mix (for biscuits or pancakes)

- 1 teaspoon Italian seasoning (or dried leaf basil and oregano)
- 1/2 teaspoon salt
- 1/2 teaspoon pepper

Instructions

1. Heat oven to 375°F (190°C) and lightly spray or oil 12 muffin cups.
2. Sprinkle cheese, onions, broccoli and tomatoes in muffin cups.
3. In a bowl, place remaining ingredients and beat until smooth. Pour egg mix over other ingredients in muffin cups.
4. Bake until golden brown, about 35-40 minutes or until knife inserted in center comes out clean. Cool 5 minutes.
5. Refrigerate leftovers.

Cheese Broccoli Mini Egg Omelettes

SERVINGS: **9**
PREP TIME: **10 min.**
TOTAL TIME: **40 min.**

Ingredients

- 4 cups broccoli florets
- 4 whole eggs
- 1 cup egg whites
- 1/4 cup reduced fat cheddar
- 1/4 cup grated Romano or parmesan cheese

- 1 tablespoon olive oil
- salt and fresh pepper
- cooking spray

Instructions

1. Preheat oven to 350°F (175°C). Steam broccoli with some water for 6-7 minutes.
2. When broccoli is cooked, mash into smaller pieces. Add olive oil, salt and pepper. Mix well.
3. Spray muffin tin with cooking spray and spoon broccoli mixture evenly into 9 tins.
4. Beat egg whites, eggs, grated parmesan cheese, salt and pepper in a medium bowl. Pour into greased tins over broccoli until a little more than 3/4 full. Top with grated cheddar and bake in the oven about 20 minutes or until cooked.
5. Serve immediately.

Peanut Butter & Banana Breakfast Smoothie
SERVINGS: **1**
PREP/TOTAL TIME: **5 min.**

Ingredients
- 1 cup non-fat milk
- 1 tablespoon all natural peanut butter
- 1 medium banana, frozen or fresh

Instructions

1. Combine all ingredients in food processor or blender. Blend until smooth.

15

Baked Apple Spice Oatmeal

SERVINGS: **9**
PREP TIME: **15 min.**
TOTAL TIME: **45 min.**

Ingredients

- 1 beaten egg
- 1/2 cup applesauce, sweetened
- 1 1/2 cups non-fat or 1% milk
- 1 teaspoon vanilla
- 2 tablespoons oil
- 1 apple, chopped (about 1 1/2 cups)
- 2 cups rolled oats
- 1 teaspoon baking powder
- 1/4 teaspoon salt
- 1 teaspoon cinnamon
- 2 tablespoons brown sugar
- 2 tablespoons chopped nuts

Instructions

1. Preheat oven to 375°F (190°C). Lightly oil or spray an 8 by 8 inch baking pan.
2. In a bowl, combine egg, applesauce, milk, vanilla, and oil. Add apple
3. In a separate bowl, mix rolled oats, baking powder, salt and cinnamon. Add to the liquid ingredients and combine well. Pour mix into baking dish and bake for 25 minutes.

4. Remove from oven and sprinkle with brown sugar and nuts. Return to oven and broil for 3 to 4 minutes or until top is browned and sugar bubbles.
5. Cut into squares and serve warm.

Strawberry Tapioca

SERVINGS: **4**
PREP TIME: **10 min.**
TOTAL TIME: **30 min.**

Ingredients

- 1/2 cup fresh strawberries, hulled and halved
- 1 1/2 cups water
- 1/4 cup quick-cooking tapioca

Instructions

1. In a food processor or in a blender blend strawberries and water until smooth. Pour into a small saucepan.
2. Add and stir in tapioca. Let stand for 10 minutes or until softened. Bring to a boil over medium heat, stir frequently to prevent sticking. Remove when thick and pour into serving dishes.

Strawberry Salad with Balsamic Vinegar

SERVINGS: **6**
PREP TIME: **10 min.**
TOTAL TIME: 1 hour 10 min.

Ingredients

- 16 ounce fresh strawberries, hulled and large berries cut in half
- 2 tablespoons balsamic vinegar
- 1/4 cup white sugar
- 1/4 teaspoon freshly ground black pepper, or to taste

Instructions

1. Place strawberries in a bowl and drizzle vinegar over strawberries. Sprinkle with sugar. Stir gently. Cover, and let sit at room temperature for between 1 and 4 hours.
2. Grind pepper over berries before serving.

Blueberry Steel Cut Oat Pancakes with Agave

SERVINGS: **10**
PREP/TOTAL TIME: **25 min.**

Ingredients

- 1 1/2 cups water
- 1/2 cup steel cut oats
- 1/8 teaspoon sea salt
- 1 cup whole wheat flour
- 1/2 teaspoon baking powder
- 1/2 teaspoon baking soda
- 1 egg
- 1 cup milk
- 1/2 cup Greek yogurt, vanilla flavor

- 1 cup frozen blueberries
- 1/2 cup + 2 tablespoons agave nectar

Instructions

1. Bring water to a boil in a medium pot and add steel cut oats and salt. Reduce heat to a simmer and cook until oats are tender, around 10 minutes. Remove from heat and set aside.
2. Combine whole wheat pastry flour, baking powder and soda, egg, milk and yogurt in a medium mixing bowl. Mix until a batter is formed. Gently fold in blueberries and cooked oats.
3. Heat non-stick skillet over medium heat and coat with cooking spray. Spoon one quarter cup of batter on surface and cook until pancakes are slightly golden, about 2-3 minutes per side.
4. Garnish each pancake with about one tablespoon agave nectar.

LUNCH

Buffalo Chicken Salad Wrap

SERVINGS: **4**
PREP TIME: **10 min.**
TOTAL TIME: **20 min.**

Ingredients

- 3-4 ounces of chicken breasts (can also use leftover or rotisserie chicken).
- 2 whole chipotle peppers
- 1/4 cup white wine vinegar
- 1/4 cup low-calorie mayonnaise
- 2 stalks celery, diced
- 2 carrots, cut into matchsticks
- 1 small yellow onion (about 1/2 cup), diced
- 1/2 cup thinly sliced rutabaga or another root vegetable
- 4 ounces spinach, cut into strips
- 2 whole-grain tortillas (12-inch diameter)

Instructions

1. If using uncooked chicken, preheat oven to 375°F (190°C) or start the grill. Bake or grill chicken breasts for 10 minutes on both sides until interior temperature is 165°F (75°C). Remove, cool and cut the chicken into cubes.
2. Puree chipotle peppers with white wine vinegar and mayonnaise in a blender. In a bowl, place all ingredients except spinach and tortillas. Mix thoroughly.
3. Place 2 ounces of spinach and half the mix in each tortilla and wrap.
4. Cut each in half to serve.

Chicken sliders

SERVINGS: **4**
PREP TIME: **10 min.**

TOTAL TIME: **1 hour**

Ingredients

- 10 ounces ground chicken breast
- 1 tablespoon black pepper
- 1 tablespoon minced garlic
- 1 tablespoon balsamic vinegar
- 1/2 cup minced onion
- 1 fresh chili pepper, minced
- 1 tablespoon fennel seed, crushed
- 4 whole wheat mini buns
- 4 lettuce leaves
- 4 tomato slices

Instructions

1. Combine and mix the first 7 items together. Let set for 1 hour.
2. Form the mix into 2-ounce patties.
3. Grill or broil in the oven until a minimum internal temperature of 165°F (75°C) is reached.
4. Serve on toasted buns with lettuce, tomatoes, and sauce of your choice.

Tuna Melt

SERVINGS: **4**
PREP TIME: **10 min.**
TOTAL TIME: **20 min.**

Ingredients

- 6 ounces white tuna packed in water, drained
- 1/3 cup chopped celery
- 1/4 cup chopped onion
- 1/4 cup low fat Russian or Thousand Island salad dressing
- 2 whole-wheat English muffins, split
- 3 ounces reduced-fat Cheddar cheese, grated
- Salt and black pepper, to taste

Instructions

1. Preheat broiler.
2. Combine tuna, celery, onion and salad dressing. Season with salt and pepper.
3. Toast English muffin halves. Place split-side-up on baking sheet and top with a quarter of tuna mixture. Broil 2-3 minutes or until heated through.
4. Top with cheese and return to broiler until cheese is melted, around 1 minute longer.

Curried Garbanzo Beans and Mustard Greens with Sweet Potatoes

SERVINGS: **4**
PREP TIME: **10 min.**
TOTAL TIME: **35 min.**

Ingredients

- 2 medium sweet potatoes, peeled and sliced thin

- 1 medium onion, cut in half and sliced thin
- 2 medium cloves garlic, sliced
- 1/2 cup + 1 tablespoons low sodium chicken or vegetable broth
- 1/2 teaspoon curry powder
- 1/4 teaspoon turmeric
- 2 cups chopped and rinsed mustard greens
- 1 (15 ounce) can sodium free diced tomatoes
- 1 (15 ounce) can garbanzo beans (chickpeas), drained and rinsed
- 2 tablespoon extra-virgin olive oil
- white pepper, to taste

Instructions

1. Steam sweet potatoes for around 5–8 minutes.
2. Heat 1 tablespoon of broth in large skillet. Sauté onion over medium heat in broth for about 4–5 minutes until translucent, stirring frequently.
3. Add garlic, curry powder, turmeric, and mustard greens. Cook, occasionally stirring until mustard greens are wilted, around 5 minutes. Add garbanzo beans, diced tomatoes, salt and pepper. Cook for another 5 minutes.
4. Mash sweet potatoes with olive oil, salt and pepper.
5. Serve mustard greens with mashed sweet potatoes.

Roasted Brussel Sprouts and Caramelized Butternut Squash with Quinoa

SERVINGS: **6**

PREP TIME: **10 min.**
TOTAL TIME: **40 min.**

Ingredients

- 1 cup quinoa, rinsed
- 2 cups low sodium chicken broth
- 9 ounces shaved Brussels sprouts
- 2 tablespoons extra virgin olive oil, divided
- Garlic powder & pepper, to taste
- 2 cups butternut squash, 1/2 inch cubed
- 1 tablespoon brown sugar
- 1/3 cup grated parmesan cheese

Instructions

1. In a saucepan bring broth to a boil then add rinsed quinoa. Cover then turn heat down to medium-low and simmer about 15 minutes or until tender. Fluff with a fork and set aside.
2. Preheat oven to 375°F (190°C) and line a baking sheet with foil. Add Brussels sprouts, 1 tablespoon oil, garlic powder, and pepper to baking sheet. Toss to evenly coat. Roast 15 minutes or until brown and golden.
3. In a large cast iron or heavy bottomed skillet, heat 1 tablespoon oil over medium-high heat. Add brown sugar and butternut squash. Sauté, stirring occasionally until tender, about 15 minutes.
4. In a large bowl combine quinoa, Brussels sprouts, butternut squash, and parmesan cheese. Toss and serve with extra parmesan cheese, if desired.

Turkey, Pear, and Cheese Sandwich

SERVINGS: **2**
PREP/TOTAL TIME: **10 min.**

Ingredients

- 2 slices multi-grain or rye sandwich bread
- 2 teaspoon Dijon-style mustard
- 2 slices (1 oz. each) reduced-sodium cooked or smoked turkey
- 1 pear, cored and thinly sliced
- 1/4 cup shredded low fat mozzarella cheese
- Coarsely ground pepper, to taste

Instructions

1. Spread each slice of bread with 1 teaspoon mustard. Place one slice turkey on each slice. Arrange pear slices on turkey. Sprinkle each with 2 tablespoons of cheese and some pepper.
2. Broil for 2 to 3 minutes, 4 to 6 inches from heat, or until turkey and pears are warm and the cheese has melted. Cut each sandwich in half and serve open face.

Salmon Salad Pita

SERVINGS: **2**
PREP/TOTAL TIME: **5 min.**

Ingredients

- 3/4 cup canned Alaskan salmon
- 3 tablespoons plain fat-free yogurt
- 1 tablespoon lemon juice
- 2 tablespoons red bell pepper, minced
- 1 tablespoon red onion, minced
- 1 teaspoon capers, rinsed and chopped
- Pinch of dill, fresh or dried
- Black pepper to taste
- 3 lettuce leaves
- 3 pieces small whole wheat pita bread

Instructions

1. Mix all ingredients together, except lettuce and pita bread, in a small bowl. Place 1 lettuce leaf and 1/3 cup salmon salad inside each pita.

Turkey Apple Gyro

SERVINGS: **6**
PREP/TOTAL TIME: **10 min.**

Ingredients

- 1 tablespoon vegetable oil
- 1 cup onion, sliced
- 1 cup sweet red pepper, thinly sliced
- 1 cup sweet green pepper, thinly sliced
- 2 tablespoons lemon juice
- 1/2 pound cooked turkey or chicken breast, cut into thin strips

- 1 Golden Delicious apple, cored and finely chopped
- 6 whole wheat pocket pita bread, warmed
- 1/2 cup low fat or fat free plain yogurt

Instructions

1. Heat oil over medium heat in a large skillet. Add onion, peppers, and lemon juice. Cook until tender.
2. Add turkey and apple and cook until turkey is heated through.
3. Remove from heat.
4. Fill each pita with some of the cooked mix.
5. Drizzle with yogurt and serve warm.

Southwest Style Rice Bowl

SERVINGS: **2**
PREP TIME: **20 min.**
TOTAL TIME: **30 min.**

Ingredients

- 1 teaspoon vegetable oil
- 1 cup chopped vegetables (bell peppers, onion, corn, tomato, zucchini, etc.)
- 1 cup cooked meat or tofu (chopped or shredded)
- 1 cup cooked brown rice
- 4 tablespoons salsa
- 2 tablespoons shredded cheese
- 2 tablespoons low fat sour cream

Instructions

1. Heat oil in a medium sized skillet over medium high heat (or 350°F (175°C) in an electric skillet). Add vegetables and cook for 3 to 5 minutes or until vegetables are tender-crisp.
2. Add cooked meat or tofu and cooked rice to skillet until heated through.
3. Divide rice mix between two bowls. Top with salsa, cheese, sour cream and serve warm.

Sunshine Wrap

SERVINGS: **4**
PREP TIME: **10 min.**
TOTAL TIME: **15 min.**

Ingredients

- 8 ounces chicken breast (one large breast)
- 1/2 cup celery, diced
- 2/3 cup canned mandarin oranges, drained
- 1/4 cup onion, minced
- 2 tablespoons mayonnaise
- 1 teaspoon soy sauce
- 1/4 teaspoon garlic powder
- 1/4 teaspoon black pepper
- 1 large whole wheat tortilla
- 4 large lettuce leaves, washed and patted dry

Instructions

1. In a non-stick pan, cook chicken breast on medium-high heat until cooked throughout (internal

temperature of 165ºF). When chicken has cooled, cut into 1/2 inch cubes.

2. Mix chicken, celery, oranges and onions in a medium bowl. Add mayonnaise, soy sauce, garlic and pepper. Mix until chicken is evenly coated.
3. Lay tortilla on large plate. With a knife or clean kitchen scissors cut tortilla into four quarters. Place 1 lettuce leaf on each tortilla quarter, trimming it so it doesn't hang over tortilla. Put 1/4 of the chicken mixture in the middle of each lettuce leaf. Roll tortillas into a cone.

Tuna Pita Pockets

SERVINGS: **6**
PREP/TOTAL TIME: **10 min.**

Ingredients
- 1 1/2 cups shredded romaine lettuce
- 3/4 cup diced tomatoes
- 1/2 cup finely chopped green bell peppers
- 1/2 cup shredded carrots
- 1/2 cup finely chopped broccoli
- 1/4 cup finely chopped onion
- 2 cans (6 ounces each) low-salt white tuna packed in water, drained
- 1/2 cup low-fat ranch dressing
- 3 whole-wheat pita pockets, cut in half

Instructions

1. Add the lettuce, tomatoes, peppers, carrots, broccoli and onions in a large bowl. Toss to mix.
2. Add tuna and ranch dressing in a small bowl. Stir to combine. Combine tuna mix with the lettuce mix.
3. Scoop 3/4 cup of the tuna salad into each pita pocket half and serve.

SALADS

Citrus Salad

SERVINGS: **4**
PREP/TOTAL TIME: **15 min.**

Ingredients
- 2 oranges
- 1 red grapefruit
- 2 tablespoons orange juice
- 2 tablespoons olive oil
- 1 tablespoon balsamic vinegar
- 4 cups spring greens
- 2 tablespoons pine nuts
- 2 tablespoons chopped mint for garnish (optional)

Instructions

1. Remove white pith and membrane of each orange and grapefruit. For each orange section remove the seeds.
2. In a bowl, combine orange juice, olive oil and vinegar. Pour mix over fruit segments and toss gently to evenly coat.
3. Divide spring greens among individual plates. Top each with the fruit and dressing mix. Sprinkle each with 1/2 tablespoon pine nuts. Garnish with chopped mint (optional).

Raw Kale Salad with Lemon Tahini Dressing
SERVINGS: **4**
> **PREP/TOTAL TIME:** 15 min. + refrigeration

Ingredients
> **Lemon Tahini Dressing:**
- Makes about 1 cup of dressing
- Ingredients:
- 3 tablespoons Tahini
- 1 tablespoon fat-free Greek Yogurt
- 2 garlic gloves
- Juice from 2 lemons, about 1/2 cup
- 1 teaspoon pepper
- Pinch of salt
- 3 tablespoons of water, or as needed
> **Salad:**
- 1/2 large head of kale, about 4-6 cups

- 1 cup finely chopped red onion
- 1 cup red bell pepper, chopped
- 1/2 cup carrot, chopped
- 1 cup cherry tomatoes, cut in half
- 1/2 cup cucumber, chopped
- 1/4 cup chopped almonds
- 1/4 cup reduced-fat shredded parmesan

Instructions

1. Add all dressing ingredients to a food processor, and blend until smooth. Set aside.
2. Wash kale under cold water and pat dry. Cut leaves from stems and chop into bite sized pieces. Place in a large bowl.
3. Top kale with chopped vegetables and walnuts. Toss.
4. Pour dressing and combine until all ingredients are covered. Top with cheese. Place in refrigerator and let marinate for about 15 minutes or cover and refrigerate for 24 hours.

Black Bean Southwest Salad

SERVINGS: **13**

    PREP/TOTAL TIME: 10 min. + refrigeration

Ingredients

- 1 can (15.5 ounce) black beans, rinsed and drained
- 9 ounce cooked corn, fresh or frozen (thawed if frozen)

- 1 medium tomato, chopped
- 1/3 cup red onion, chopped
- 1 scallion, chopped
- 2 limes, juice of
- 1 tablespoon olive oil
- 2 tablespoon fresh minced cilantro
- 1 teaspoon salt
- 1 teaspoon fresh black pepper
- 1/2 medium hass avocado, diced
- 1/4 cup queso fresco (cotija) cheese
- 1 diced jalapeno (optional)

Instructions

1. Combine beans, corn, tomato, onion, scallion, cilantro, salt and pepper in a large bowl. Squeeze fresh lime juice to taste and stir in olive oil. Marinate in the refrigerator 30 minutes.
2. Add avocado and cheese before serving.

Mediterranean Tuna Salad
SERVINGS: 10
PREP/TOTAL TIME: 5 min.

Ingredients

- 3 cans (5 ounces each) tuna in water, drained
- 1 cup shredded carrot
- 2 cups diced cucumber
- 1 1/2 cups peas, canned and drained or thawed from frozen

- 3/4 cup low-fat, low-sodium Italian salad dressing

Instructions

1. Place drained tuna in a medium bowl. Break apart chunks with a fork. Add carrot, cucumber, peas and salad dressing. Mixing well.
2. Serve immediately or cover and refrigerate until ready to serve.

Tangy Mango Salad

SERVINGS: **6**
PREP/TOTAL TIME: **10 min.**

Ingredients

- 3 ripe mangoes, pitted and cubed
- Juice of 1 lime
- 1 teaspoon minced red onion
- 2 tablespoons chopped fresh cilantro leaves
- Half of 1 jalapeno pepper, seeded and minced

Instructions

1. Combine all ingredients in a mixing bowl and let stand 10 minutes.
2. Toss before serving.

Winter Citrus Salad

SERVINGS: **6**
PREP/TOTAL TIME: **10 min.**

Ingredients

- 8 cups mixed greens (spinach, arugula, red leaf lettuce)
- 2 ruby red grapefruits, peeled and cut into sections
- 2 navel oranges, peeled and cut into sections
- 1/2 avocado, cubed
- 1/4 cup sliced almonds, toasted
- 2 ounces Asiago cheese, shaved
- 4 tablespoons of your favorite balsamic vinaigrette dressing

Instructions

1. Toss ingredients together in a large salad bowl.
2. Serve.

Pineapple Chicken Salad with Balsamic Vinaigrette

SERVINGS: 8

PREP TIME: **5 min.**
TOTAL TIME: **15 min.**

Ingredients

- 4 boneless, skinless chicken breasts (5 ounces each)
- 1 tablespoon olive oil
- 1 can (8 ounces) unsweetened pineapple chunks, drained (set aside 2 tablespoons of juice)
- 2 cups broccoli florets
- 4 cups fresh baby spinach leaves

- 1/2 cup thinly sliced red onions
- 1/4 cup olive oil
- 2 tablespoons balsamic vinegar
- 2 teaspoons sugar
- 1/4 teaspoon ground cinnamon

Instructions

1. Cut each chicken breast into cubes. Heat olive oil over medium heat in a large, non-stick frying pan. Add chicken and cook until golden brown, about 10 minutes.
2. In a large serving bowl, combine cooked chicken, pineapple chunks, broccoli, spinach and onions.
3. In a small bowl, whisk together the olive oil, vinegar, reserved pineapple juice, sugar and cinnamon. Pour over the salad and gently toss to coat. Serve immediately.

Grilled Chicken Avocado and Mango Salad
SERVINGS: 4
PREP/TOTAL TIME: 7 min.

Ingredients

- 12 ounce grilled chicken breast, sliced
- 1 cup diced avocado
- 1 cup diced mango
- 2 tablespoons diced red onion
- 6 cups baby red butter lettuce
- 2 tablespoons olive oil

- 2 tablespoons white balsamic vinegar

Instructions

1. Whisk olive oil and balsamic vinegar together. Set aside.
2. Toss together avocado, mango, chicken, and red onion.
3. Fill a large salad platter with baby greens or divide them amongst four plates.
4. Top greens with chicken and avocado mix.
5. Drizzle vinegar dressing among the four servings.

Southwestern Black Bean Cakes with Guacamole

SERVINGS: **4**
PREP TIME: **10 min.**
TOTAL TIME: **20 min.**

Ingredients

- 2 slices whole wheat bread, torn
- 3 tablespoons fresh cilantro
- 2 cloves garlic
- 1 can (15-ounce) low sodium black beans, rinsed and drained
- 1 can (7-ounce) chipotle peppers in adobo sauce
- 1 teaspoon ground cumin
- 1 large egg
- 1/2 medium avocado, seeded and peeled
- 1 tablespoon lime juice

- 1 small plum tomato

Instructions

1. Place torn bread in a blender. Cover and blend until bread turns into coarse crumbs. Transfer to a large bowl and set aside.
2. Process cilantro and garlic until finely chopped. Add beans, 1 of the chipotle peppers, 1 to 2 teaspoons of adobo sauce, and cumin. Process by pulsing in a blender until beans are coarsely chopped and mix pull away from sides.
3. Add mix to bread crumbs in bowl. Add egg and combine well.
4. Shape mixture into four 1/2-inch-thick patties. Grill directly over medium heat for 8 to 10 minutes or until patties are heated through, turning once.
5. To make guacamole, mash avocado in small bowl. Stir in lime juice and season with salt and pepper. Serve patties with guacamole and tomato.

Almond Chicken Pear Salad
SERVINGS: 4
PREP/ TOTAL TIME: **5 min.**

Ingredients

- 2 cups cooked boneless, skinless, chicken breasts, cut in 1/2-inch cubes
- 1/2 cup green pepper, sliced lengthwise
- 1/4 cup diced celery
- 1/4 teaspoon salt

- 1/2 cup low-fat plain yogurt
- 2 tablespoons reduced-calorie mayonnaise
- 1/2 teaspoon prepared mustard
- 1/4 teaspoon ground ginger
- 2 fresh Pears, cored and cut in 1-inch cubes
- Favorite lettuce
- 2 tablespoons toasted slivered almonds

Instructions

1. Toss together chicken, green pepper and celery. Sprinkle with salt.
2. Combine yogurt, mayonnaise, mustard and ginger. Add to chicken mixture.
3. Add in the pears to the mixture.
4. Serve on individual lettuce-lined salad plates and sprinkle with almonds.

Curried Garbanzo Beans and Mustard Greens with Sweet Potatoes

SERVINGS: **4**
PREP TIME: **10 min.**
TOTAL TIME: **35 min.**

Ingredients

- 2 medium sweet potatoes, peeled and sliced thin
- 1 medium onion, cut in half and sliced thin
- 2 medium cloves garlic, sliced
- 1/2 cup + 1 tablespoons low sodium vegetable broth

- 1/2 teaspoon curry powder
- 1/4 teaspoon turmeric
- 2 cups chopped and rinsed mustard greens
- 1 (15 ounce) can sodium free diced tomatoes
- 1 (15 ounce) can garbanzo beans (chickpeas), drained and rinsed
- 2 tablespoon extra-virgin olive oil
- white pepper, to taste

Instructions

1. Steam sweet potatoes for around 5–8 minutes.
2. Heat 1 tablespoon of broth in large skillet. Sauté onion over medium heat in broth for about 4–5 minutes until translucent, stirring frequently.
3. Add garlic, curry powder, turmeric, and mustard greens. Cook, occasionally stirring until mustard greens are wilted, around 5 minutes. Add garbanzo beans, diced tomatoes, salt and pepper. Cook for another 5 minutes.
4. Mash sweet potatoes with olive oil, salt and pepper.
5. Serve mustard greens with mashed sweet potatoes.

Mango Curry Chicken Salad
SERVINGS: 4
PREP/TOTAL TIME: 7 min.

Ingredients

- 2 1/2 cups (1/2 inch pieces) grilled skinless, boneless chicken breasts

- 3/4 cup plain, non-fat yogurt
- 1 teaspoon curry
- 1/4 cup cubed mango
- 1 cup dried, sweetened cranberries
- 1/4 cup walnuts, coarsely chopped
- 1/3 cup Mozzarella cheese, cut into small cubes

Instructions

1. In a medium bowl, whisk yogurt and curry together. Stir in chicken, mango, cranberries, walnuts and Mozzarella cheese.
2. Mix well and serve on lettuce leaves, if desired.

Avocado Salad with Ginger-Miso Dressing
SERVINGS: **6**

  PREP/TOTAL TIME: 15 min. + refrigeration

Ingredients
- 1/3 cup plain silken tofu
- 1/3 cup low-fat plain soy milk (soya milk)
- 1 tablespoon peeled and minced fresh ginger
- 1 1/2 teaspoons reduced-sodium soy sauce
- 1 teaspoon light miso
- 1 teaspoon Dijon mustard
- 1 tablespoon chopped fresh cilantro (fresh coriander)
- 1 tablespoon chopped green (spring) onion, including tender green top

- 1 small avocado, pitted, peeled and cut into 12 thin slices
- 1 tablespoon fresh lemon juice
- 12 ounces mixed baby lettuces
- 1/4 cup chopped red onion
- 1 green (spring) onion, including tender green top, thinly sliced on the diagonal
- 1 tablespoon chopped fresh cilantro (fresh coriander)

Instructions

1. In a blender or food processor add tofu, soy milk, ginger, soy sauce, miso and mustard. Process until smooth and creamy. Transfer to a bowl and stir in the cilantro and green onion. Cover and refrigerate for at least 1 hour.
2. Toss avocado slices in the lemon juice in a small bowl. Set aside.
3. Combine the lettuces, red and green onions, and cilantro in a large bowl. Toss to mix.
4. Add 2/3 of the dressing and toss to coat. Divide salad among individual plates.
5. Arrange 2 avocado slices on top of each portion in a crisscross pattern. Top each avocado cross with a spoonful of remaining dressing. Serve immediately.

Spring Nicoise Potato Salad

SERVINGS: **4**
PREP TIME: **10 min.**
TOTAL TIME: **20 min.**

Ingredients

- 8 small red potatoes
- 1 can (6-ounce) white tuna in water, drained
- 12 steamed asparagus spears
- 8 radishes
- 9 pitted Kalamata olives
- 2 tablespoons minced red onion
- 3 tablespoons red wine vinegar
- 2 tablespoons chopped fresh parsley
- 4 teaspoons olive oil
- Black pepper, to taste

Instructions

1. Wash potatoes and leave skins on. Cut into quarters and place in large pot filled with enough water to cover potatoes. Set heat to high and bring water to boil. Boil potatoes for 10 minutes or until tender. Drain water.
2. Place potatoes on platter with tuna, asparagus, radishes, olives and onion.
3. Whisk vinegar, parsley, and oil in small bowl. Drizzle mix over the salad. Add salt and pepper, to taste.

Strawberries, Blue Cheese, and Chicken Mixed Greens Salad with Poppy Seed Dressing

SERVINGS: **4**
PREP TIME: **15 min.**
TOTAL TIME: **20 min.**

Ingredients

Dressing:

- 1 tablespoon red wine vinegar
- 1 tablespoon cider vinegar
- 2 tablespoons olive oil
- 1 teaspoon minced shallots
- 1 1/2 tablespoon honey
- 1/2 tablespoon poppy seeds

Salad:

- 5 ounces mixed baby greens
- 1/4 cup slivered almonds
- 2 cups sliced strawberries
- 1/4 cup blue cheese
- 12 ounces grilled chicken, sliced

Instructions

1. Place all salad dressing ingredients in a small jar and mix well.
2. Combine all of the salad ingredients in a large bowl.
3. Add dressing to the large bowl and toss salad until the dressing is evenly mixed.
4. Divide evenly among four plates.

Shrimp, Strawberry and Feta Salad
SERVINGS: 4

PREP TIME: **5 min.**
TOTAL TIME: **10 min.**

Ingredients

- 3 tablespoons extra virgin olive oil
- 2 tablespoons balsamic vinegar
- 2 tablespoons water
- 1/4 teaspoon salt
- 1/4 teaspoon black pepper
- 1/3 cup thinly sliced red onion
- 3/4 pound peeled and deveined raw shrimp
- 2 cups (about 10 ounces) fresh strawberries, stemmed and quartered
- 8 cups mixed salad greens, such as butter lettuce and watercress
- 2 ounces crumbled feta cheese
- 1 small cucumber, sliced (about 24 slices)

Instructions

1. In small bowl, combine olive oil and balsamic vinegar to make vinaigrette.
2. In a large bowl, toss onion with 1 tablespoon of the vinaigrette. Set aside.
3. Grill shrimp for 5 minutes until pink and cooked through, turning once, over a grill or in a pan on stove top.
4. In another small bowl, toss strawberries with 1 tablespoon of the vinaigrette.
5. Toss greens with sliced onions and enough remaining vinaigrette to lightly coat. Divide among 4 chilled salad plates and arrange strawberries and

shrimp on top of greens. Sprinkle with cheese and garnish with slices of cucumber, dividing equally.
6. Drizzle any remaining vinaigrette over salad.

Apricot Chicken Pasta Salad
SERVINGS: 4

PREP TIME: **7 min.**
TOTAL TIME: **20 min.**

Ingredients

Dressing
- 2 apricots cut into quarters
- 2 tablespoons white wine vinegar
- 1/4 teaspoon salt
- 1 tablespoon sugar
- 3 tablespoons olive oil
- 1 tablespoon finely chopped fresh basil

Salad
- 1/4 lb. fusilli (corkscrew) pasta
- 6 fresh apricots cut into quarters
- 2 cups low sodium chicken broth
- 2 skinless, boneless chicken breasts
- 1 red bell pepper cut into long thin strips
- 2 small zucchini ends trimmed, cut in half then into thin strips
- 1 tablespoon chopped fresh basil
- 1 cup apricot basil dressing

Instructions

1. In a blender, combine apricots, white wine vinegar, salt and sugar until well blended. With blender running, slowly add olive oil until thick and smooth. Stir in fresh basil.
2. Bring chicken broth to a boil in a small saucepan. Reduce heat to a simmer and add chicken breasts. Cover pan and continue to simmer until chicken is cooked through, about 6 minutes. Remove chicken from the broth. Allow to cool slightly and shred into bite sized pieces with a fork.
3. Cook pasta according to package directions. Drain and let cool. In a large bowl, combine pasta, apricots, chicken, zucchini, red pepper and basil. Toss lightly with the dressing.

Crispy Citrus Salad with Grilled Cod
SERVINGS: 2

PREP TIME: **5 min.**
TOTAL TIME: **15 min.**

Ingredients
- 6 ounces baked or broiled cod
- 1 1/2 tablespoons olive oil
- 1 1/2 cups shredded spinach
- 1 1/2 cups shredded kohlrabi
- 1 cup shredded celery
- 1 1/2 cups shredded carrot
- 2 tablespoons shredded fresh basil
- 1 tablespoon minced fresh parsley

- 3/4 cup chopped red bell pepper
- 1 teaspoon black pepper
- 1 tablespoon minced garlic
- Zest and juice of 1 lemon
- Zest and juice of 1 lime
- Zest and juice of 1 orange
- 1 cup grapefruit segments
- 1/2 cup orange segments

Instructions

1. Spray a grill or broiler pan with cooking spray. Turn on grill or preheat broiler.
2. Place cod on grill or broiler pan and brush lightly with oil. Grill or broil 3 to 4 inches from heat until fish flakes easily with a fork, about 10 minutes. If using a food thermometer, fish should reach 145°F (65°C).
3. Toss remaining ingredients together in large bowl, except for grapefruit and orange segments and cod.
4. Divide salad between two plates. Top with cod and citrus pieces.

Cinnamon Pistachio Chicken Salad
SERVINGS: 6
PREP/TOTAL TIME: 5 min.

Ingredients

- 16 ounces cooked boneless, skinless chicken breast
- 1 1/2 cups fat-free plain Greek yogurt

- 1/2 cup pistachios, finely chopped
- 1 teaspoon ground cinnamon
- 1 teaspoon fresh lime juice
- 4 fresh basil leaves, finely chopped
- 1/4 teaspoon ground pepper
- 2 scallions, finely chopped

Instructions

1. Shred cooked chicken breast with a fork. Place in a large mixing bowl.
2. Add remaining ingredients and gently toss to combine.
3. Served chilled or at room temperature.

Rocket and Veggie Ham Salad

SERVINGS: **2**
PREP/ TOTAL TIME: **5 min.**

Ingredients

- 1 (7 ounce) bag arugula
- 7 ounces of your favorite ham deli slices, torn into thin strips
- 1/4 cup olive oil
- 1/4 cup balsamic vinegar

Instructions

1. Place arugula on a large flat platter.
2. Top with ham.
3. Drizzle olive oil and balsamic vinegar on top.

SOUPS

Ginger Chicken Noodle Soup
SERVINGS: 8

PREP TIME: **10 min.**
TOTAL TIME: **20 min.**

Ingredients
- 3 ounces dried soba noodles
- 1 tablespoon olive oil
- 1 large yellow onion, chopped
- 1 tablespoon peeled and minced fresh ginger
- 1 carrot, peeled and finely chopped
- 1 clove garlic, minced
- 4 cups chicken stock or broth
- 2 tablespoons reduced-sodium soy sauce
- 1 pound skinless, boneless chicken breasts, chopped
- 1 cup shelled edamame
- 1 cup plain soy milk
- 1/4 cup chopped fresh cilantro/coriander

Instructions
1. Boil a saucepan 3/4 full of water. Add noodles and cook until tender, about 5 minutes. Drain and set aside.
2. Heat olive oil over medium heat in a large saucepan. Add onion and sauté about 4 minutes or until soft and translucent. Add ginger and carrot and sauté for

1 minute. Add garlic and sauté for 30 seconds, not letting garlic brown. Add in stock and soy sauce and bring to a boil. Add the chicken and edamame. Reduce the heat after boiling to medium-low and simmer until chicken is cooked and the edamame are tender, about 4 minutes. Add soba noodles and soy milk and cook until heated through, without letting it boil.

3. Remove pan from heat and stir in the cilantro. Ladle soup into individual bowls and serve.

Autumn Squash Ginger Bisque

SERVINGS: **5**
PREP TIME: **10 min.**
TOTAL TIME: **1 hour**

Ingredients
- 2 teaspoons vegetable oil
- 2 cups sliced onions
- 2 pounds winter squash, peeled, seeded, and cut into 2-inch cubes (about 4 cups)
- 2 pears, peeled, cored, and diced, or 1 can (15 ounces) sliced pears in juice, drained and chopped
- 2 cloves garlic, peeled and crushed
- 2 tablespoons coarsely chopped, peeled fresh ginger, or 1 teaspoon powdered ginger
- 1/2 teaspoon thyme
- 4 cups low-sodium chicken or vegetable broth
- 1 cup water

- 1 tablespoon lemon juice
- 1/2 cup plain non-fat yogurt

Instructions

1. In a large pot heat oil over medium heat. Add onions and cook for 3 to 4 minutes, stirring constantly until softened. Add squash, pears, garlic, ginger and thyme. Cook for 1 minute while stirring.
2. Add broth and water and bring to a simmer. Reduce heat to low. Cover and simmer 35-45 minutes or until squash is tender.
3. Puree soup in a food processor or blender, in batches if necessary. (Follow manufacturer's directions for pureeing hot liquids if using a blender). Return soup to pot and heat. Stir in lemon juice.
4. Garnish each serving with a dollop of yogurt.

Potato Soup with Brie Cheese and Apple

SERVINGS: **8**
PREP TIME: **15 min.**
TOTAL TIME: **1 hour**

Ingredients

- 1 cup chopped yellow onion
- 1/4 cup sliced leeks (whites only)
- 4 large Granny Smith apples, cored, peeled and quartered

- 1 Granny Smith apple, cored and sliced thinly, for garnish
- 2 cups low-sodium chicken broth
- 1 bay leaf
- 1/4 teaspoon dried thyme
- 3 cups fat-free evaporated milk
- 6 small potatoes, peeled and sliced
- 4 ounces brie cheese, cut into small cubes

Instructions

1. Spray a soup pot with cooking spray. Add onion, leeks and 4 apples. Sauté 5 to 7 minutes over medium heat until softened. Add broth, bay leaf, and thyme. Bring to a boil, reduce heat to low and simmer for 15 minutes. Remove bay leaf. Turn off heat and set the mix aside.
2. While the broth mix is cooking, combine evaporated milk and potatoes in a separate saucepan. Cook over medium heat 15 to 20 minutes until potatoes are tender. Stir frequently. Pour potato mix into soup pot. Stir to evenly mix.
3. In a blender or food processor, puree the soup in batches until smooth, adding pieces of brie cheese during pureeing. Return pureed batch to the soup pot and heat until heated through.
4. Ladle into individual bowls and garnish with thin slices of apple.

Greek Lentil Soup

SERVINGS: **4**
PREP TIME: **20 min.**
TOTAL TIME: 1 hour 20 min

Ingredients

- 8 ounces brown lentils
- 1/4 cup olive oil
- 1 tablespoon minced garlic
- 1 onion, minced
- 1 large carrot, chopped
- 1 quart water
- 1 pinch dried oregano
- 1 pinch crushed dried rosemary
- 2 bay leaves
- 1 tablespoon tomato paste
- salt and ground black pepper, to taste
- 1 teaspoon olive oil, or to taste
- 1 teaspoon red wine vinegar, to taste

Instructions

1. Place lentils in a large saucepan. Add enough water to cover lentils by an inch. Bring water to a boil and cook about 10 minutes or until tender. Drain.
2. Heat olive oil in a saucepan over medium heat. Add garlic, onion, and carrot. Cook and stir about 5 minutes or until the onion has softened and turned translucent. Pour in lentils, 1 quart water, oregano, rosemary, and bay leaves. Bring to a boil and then reduce heat to medium-low. Cover and simmer for 10 minutes.

3. Stir in tomato paste and season with salt and pepper. Cover and simmer 30 to 40 minutes or until the lentils have softened, occasionally stirring. Add additional water if the soup becomes too thick. Drizzle with 1 teaspoon olive oil and red wine vinegar to taste.

Leftover Turkey Chili
SERVINGS: 6

PREP TIME: **10 min.**
TOTAL TIME: **25 min.**

Ingredients

- 1 tablespoon olive oil
- 2 tablespoons diced onion
- 2 teaspoon diced garlic
- 1 can (15 ounce) low sodium black beans
- 1 cup shredded precooked white meat turkey
- 3 tablespoons roasted red pepper, canned in water, drained
- 1 can (32 ounces) roasted diced tomato with juice
- 1/2 tablespoon chili powder
- 1 tablespoon cumin
- 1/2 teaspoon red pepper flakes
- 1/2 teaspoon salt
- 6 tablespoons plain fat-free yogurt
- 6 tablespoon shredded cheddar cheese

Instructions

1. Heat oil over medium heat in a large pot. Add onions and garlic and sauté about 3-4 minutes, or until onions are translucent. Add remaining ingredients, except yogurt and cheese and stir thoroughly to combine.
2. Bring chili to a simmer. Cover and let cook for 10-15 minutes.
3. Once chili is done, remove from heat.
4. Serve topped with 1 tablespoon yogurt and 1 tablespoon shredded cheddar cheese.

Roasted Pear and Squash Soup

SERVINGS: **6**
PREP TIME: **15 min.**
TOTAL TIME: **1 hour**

Ingredients

- 2 pounds Delicata Squash or Butternut Squash, cut in half lengthwise and seeded
- 2 tablespoons olive oil
- 2 firm but ripe Anjou or Bartlett pears, cut in half lengthwise and cored
- 4 cups canned low-sodium chicken broth
- 1/4 teaspoon freshly grated nutmeg
- 1 tablespoon sugar
- 1/4 teaspoon pepper
- 1/2 cup fat free evaporated milk

Instructions

1. Preheat the oven to 350°F (175°C).
2. Brush flesh of the squash and pears with olive oil. Place cut side down on a rimmed baking sheet. Place in preheated oven and roast about 30 to 35 minutes or until tender when pierced with a fork.
3. Use a spoon to scrape out the flesh of the squash and pears and place in a blender. Discard skins. Add 1 to 2 cups of the chicken broth and blend until smooth.
4. Place mixture in a 3 1/2-to 4-quart saucepan. Add remaining chicken broth, nutmeg, sugar, and pepper.
5. Bring to a boil, and then reduce to a simmer. Cook for 10 minutes. Stir in the evaporated milk and simmer until just heated through.

Curried Carrot Soup

SERVINGS: **6**
PREP TIME: **10 min.**
TOTAL TIME: **25 min.**

Ingredients
- 1 tablespoon olive oil
- 1 teaspoon mustard seed
- 1/2 yellow onion, chopped
- 1 pound carrots, peeled and cut into 1/2-inch pieces
- 1 tablespoon plus 1 teaspoon peeled and chopped fresh ginger
- 1/2 jalapeno chili, seeded

- 2 teaspoons curry powder
- 5 cups chicken stock, vegetable stock or broth
- 1/4 cup chopped fresh cilantro (fresh coriander), plus leaves for garnish
- 2 tablespoons fresh lime juice
- 1/2 teaspoon salt (optional)
- 3 tablespoons low-fat sour cream or fat-free plain yogurt
- Grated zest of 1 lime

Instructions

1. Heat olive oil over medium heat in a large saucepan. Add the mustard seed. When seeds begin to pop (about 1 minute) add onion and sauté about 4 minutes or until soft and translucent. Add carrots, ginger, jalapeno and curry powder and sauté about 3 minutes or until seasonings are fragrant.
2. Add 3 cups of the stock and raise heat to high. Bring to a boil. Reduce heat to medium-low and simmer about 6 minutes or until carrots are tender.
3. Puree soup in batches in a blender or food processor until smooth. Return to the saucepan. Stir in remaining 2 cups stock. Return soup to medium heat and reheat.
4. Just before serving, stir in chopped cilantro and lime juice. Season with the salt, if desired.
5. Garnish with a drizzle of yogurt, a sprinkle of lime zest and cilantro leaves.

Wild Rice Mushroom Soup

SERVINGS: **4**
PREP TIME: **10 min.**
TOTAL TIME: **35 min.**

Ingredients

- 1 tablespoon olive oil
- half a white onion, chopped
- 1/4 cup chopped celery
- 1/4 cup chopped carrots
- 1 1/2 cups sliced fresh white mushrooms
- 1/2 cup white wine, or 1/2 cup low-sodium, fat-free chicken broth
- 2 1/2 cups low-sodium, fat-free chicken broth
- 1 cup fat-free half-and-half
- 2 tablespoons flour
- 1/4 teaspoon dried thyme
- black pepper
- 1 cup cooked wild rice

Instructions

1. Heat olive oil in pot on medium heat. Add chopped onion, celery and carrots. Cook until tender. Add mushrooms, white wine and chicken broth. Cover until heated through.
2. Blend half-and-half, flour, thyme and pepper in a bowl. Stir in cooked wild rice. Pour rice mix into hot pot with vegetables. Cook over medium heat. Stir continually until bubbly and thickened.
3. Serve warm.

Seafood Chowder
SERVINGS: 6

PREP TIME: **10 min.**
TOTAL TIME: **40 min.**

Ingredients

- 2 medium potatoes, cubed
- 1 carrot, sliced 1/4 inch thick
- 1 medium onion, chopped
- 1 cup clam juice
- 1 cup water
- 1 tablespoon butter
- 1/4 teaspoon salt
- 1/4 teaspoon pepper
- 1 pound lean fish (halibut, cod, or salmon) cut into 1-inch pieces
- 1 can (6 1/2 ounce) clams, un-drained
- 1 can (12 ounce) evaporated skim milk
- 2 tablespoons chopped fresh chives
- 1 teaspoon paprika

Instructions

1. Combine potatoes, carrots, onion, clam juice, water, butter, salt and pepper in a large saucepan. Bring to a boil. Reduce heat, cover, and simmer 15-20 minutes or until potatoes are almost tender.
2. Stir in fish and clams, and increase heat until soup begins to boil. Reduce heat and simmer 5 minutes or until fish flakes easily with a fork.

3. Stir in milk, chives, and paprika and heat through.
4. Serve.

Spicy Chili Soup

SERVINGS: **8**
PREP TIME: **10 min.**
TOTAL TIME: **35 min.**

Ingredients

- 2 tablespoons olive oil
- 1 pound boneless skinless chicken breast, cubed
- 1 heaping tablespoon garlic, minced
- 1 medium onion, diced
- 1 bell pepper, diced
- 2 large carrots, sliced
- 1/3 cup chili powder
- 1 15 oz. can reduced sodium kidney beans, with liquid
- 2 cans no salt added diced tomatoes, with juice
- 2 cans 50% reduced sodium chicken or beef broth
- Pepper, to taste
- 1/4 teaspoon salt (optional)

Instructions

1. Sauté the cubed chicken breast in the olive oil over medium heat in a large pot, until the chicken has browned on both sides. Remove the chicken and set aside.

2. In the same pot, add in garlic, onion, bell pepper, and carrots. Sauté about 5 minutes until lightly browned, stirring occasionally. Add chili powder to the vegetable mix and sauté another 2-3 minutes.
3. Add the kidney beans with liquid, diced tomatoes with juice, broth, and cooked chicken. Bring the liquid to a simmer for 10-15 minutes or until vegetables are soft.
4. Add salt and pepper if desired. Serve hot.

Shamrock Soup

SERVINGS: **4**
PREP TIME: **15 min.**
TOTAL TIME: **45 min.**

Ingredients

- 1/2 cup each: chopped onion, carrot and celery
- 1 tablespoon butter
- 3/4 cup dry split peas, rinsed and drained
- 1 can (13 3/4 ounces) chicken broth
- 1 1/2 cups fat free milk, divided
- 4 cups washed and dried fresh spinach leaves
- 4 tablespoons diced fully cooked lean ham
- Salt and freshly ground pepper to taste
- Pinch of freshly grated or ground nutmeg

Instructions

1. In a medium saucepan, sauté onion, carrot and celery in butter until onion is soft. Add split peas,

chicken broth and half of milk. Bring to a boil, cover and reduce heat to low. Simmer for 30 minutes, occasionally stirring, until split peas are tender. Remove from heat and cool slightly.

2. Puree split pea mixture with spinach in blender or food processor. Return mix to saucepan. Stir in remaining milk until desired consistency. Cook and stir over low heat until mix comes to a simmer. Season to taste with freshly ground pepper and nutmeg.

3. Serve and sprinkle with ham.

Steamy Salmon Chowder
SERVINGS: 8

PREP TIME: **10 min.**
TOTAL TIME: **30 min.**

Ingredients

- 1 teaspoon olive oil
- 1/2 cup chopped celery
- 1 clove garlic, minced
- 1 can (15-ounce) reduced-sodium chicken broth
- 2 1/2 cups frozen country-style hash browns with green pepper and onion
- 1 cup frozen peas and carrots
- 1/2 teaspoon dill
- 1/2 teaspoon ground pepper
- 6 ounces pouched or canned pink salmon, with bones removed

- 1 can (12-ounce) evaporated skim milk
- 1 can (14 3/4 ounces) no-salt-added, cream-style corn

Instructions

1. In a large saucepan over medium heat, sauté olive oil and celery for 10 minutes. Add garlic and sauté another minute.
2. Add the chicken broth, hash browns, peas and carrots, dill and pepper and bring to a boil. Reduce heat and simmer for about 10 minutes, until the vegetables are cooked.
3. Add salmon, separating into pieces with a fork. Stir in evaporated milk and corn and cook until heated through.

DINNER

Grilled Pineapple Salsa Beef Kabobs
SERVINGS: 6

PREP TIME: **15 min.**
TOTAL TIME: **30 min. + margination**

Ingredients

- 1-1/2 pounds beef shoulder center (Ranch) steaks, cut 1 inch thick
- Salt and pepper

  Marinade:

- 2 tablespoons fresh lime juice
- 2 tablespoons olive oil
- 2 large cloves garlic, minced
- 1 medium jalapeno pepper, minced
- 1/2 teaspoon ground cumin

Pineapple Salsa:
- 1/2 medium pineapple (about 3 cups), peeled, cored, cut into 1-1/2 inch chunks
- 1 medium red onion, cut into 12 wedges
- 1 large red or green bell pepper, cut into 1-1/2 inch pieces
- 2 teaspoons freshly grated lime peel
- 1/2 teaspoon salt

Instructions

1. Cut beef steaks in 1-1/4-inch pieces. In a medium bowl, combine marinade ingredients. Reserve 2 tablespoons of marinade for salsa. Add beef to remaining marinade and toss to coat. Cover and marinate 30 minutes to 2 hours in refrigerator.
2. Remove beef from marinade. Place beef pieces onto six 10-inch metal skewers, leaving small space between pieces, or place fruit and vegetable pieces evenly on six 10-inch metal skewers.
3. Place fruit and vegetable kabobs on a grill over medium, ash-covered coals. Grill uncovered for 12 to 15 minutes, until vegetables are tender, occasionally turn. Remove and keep warm. Place beef kabobs in the center of grid. Grill covered, for 7

to 9 minutes until medium rare to medium doneness, occasionally turning.

4. Remove fruit and vegetables from skewers and coarsely chop. In a medium bowl, combine with reserved marinade, lime peel, and 1/2 teaspoon salt.

5. Season beef with salt and pepper, as desired. Serve with Pineapple Salsa.

Sesame-Honey Chicken and Quinoa
SERVINGS: 4

PREP TIME: **10 min.**
TOTAL TIME: **35 min.**

Ingredients

- 1 1/2 cups water
- 3/4 cup quinoa, rinsed
- 2 cups grated carrots (about 3 large sized)
- 2 tablespoons rice vinegar
- 2 tablespoons sesame seeds, toasted
- 1 tablespoon sesame oil
- 2 tablespoons sesame oil
- 2 cups cooked chicken breast, cut into bite-sized pieces
- 3 tablespoons honey
- 3 tablespoons reduced-sodium soy sauce
- 2 tablespoons water
- 1 teaspoon corn-starch
- 2 scallions, sliced

Instructions

1. Bring 1 1/2 cups water to a boil in a small saucepan. Add quinoa and return to a boil. Reduce to a simmer, cover and cook until the water is absorbed, around 10 to 14 minutes. Uncover and let stand.
2. In a medium bowl, combine carrots, rice vinegar, sesame seeds, and 1 tablespoon oil. Set aside.
3. In a small bowl, combine sesame oil, honey, soy sauce, 2 tablespoons water and corn-starch. Pour into a medium skillet. Cook over medium heat, and stir until sauce has thickened. Add chicken and stir until coated with sauce, about 1 minute.
4. Divide quinoa among 4 bowls and top each with 1/2 cup carrot slaw and 3/4 cup chicken mix. Sprinkle with scallions.

Shrimp Pasta Primavera
SERVINGS: 6

PREP TIME: **10 min.**
TOTAL TIME: **30 min.**

Ingredients

- 1-1/4 cup fresh asparagus, sliced into 1 inch lengths (about 1/2 pound)
- 12 ounces whole wheat penne pasta
- 1 cup green peas, fresh or frozen
- 2 teaspoon olive oil
- 1 tablespoon garlic, minced
- 1/8 teaspoon crushed red pepper

- 1 pound medium shrimp, peeled and deveined
- 1/2 cup green onion, thinly sliced
- 2 teaspoon fresh lemon juice
- 1 tablespoon fresh parsley, chopped
- 1/3 cup grated Parmesan cheese
- 1/2 teaspoon salt
- Fresh ground black pepper

Instructions

1. Boil a 6 quart pot of water. Add asparagus and cook until tender-crisp, around 4 minutes. Transfer to a bowl. Add pasta and cook according to the package directions. In the last 2 minutes of cooking, add peas. Drain pasta with the peas and reserve in the bowl with the asparagus.
2. Heat olive oil over medium heat in a 12-inch non-stick skillet. Add minced garlic and crushed red pepper. Cook and stir until fragrant, about 1 minute. Add shrimp and cook for 2 minutes on each side. Add pasta with the vegetables, green onion, lemon juice, parsley and Parmesan cheese. Toss to coat and season with salt and fresh ground black pepper, to taste.

Chicken Pesto Bake
SERVINGS: 4

PREP TIME: **5 min.**
TOTAL TIME: **25 min.**

Ingredients

- 2 boneless, skinless chicken breasts (160 total ounces)
- 4 teaspoons basil pesto
- 1 medium tomato, sliced thin
- 6 tablespoons shredded reduced fat mozzarella cheese
- 2 teaspoons grated parmesan cheese

Instructions

1. Wash chicken and pat dry with paper towel. Slice chicken breast horizontally to create 4 thin pieces.
2. Preheat the oven to 400°F (200°C). Line a baking sheet with foil or parchment.
3. Place chicken on the baking sheet and spread 1 teaspoon of pesto on chicken piece.
4. Bake until chicken is no longer pink in the center, about 15 minutes. Remove from oven and top with tomatoes, mozzarella, and parmesan cheese.
5. Return to oven for another 3 to 5 minutes or until the cheese melts.

Grilled Chicken with Crunchy Apple Salsa
SERVINGS: 4

PREP TIME: **15 min.**

TOTAL TIME: 35 min. + refrigeration

Ingredients

- 2 cups chopped, cored Gala apples
- 1 Anaheim chili pepper, seeded and chopped

- 1/2 cup chopped onion
- 1/4 cup lime juice
- salt and black pepper
- 1/4 cup dry white wine
- 1/4 cup apple juice
- 1/2 teaspoon grated lime zest
- 1/2 teaspoon salt
- 1/8 teaspoon black pepper
- 2 whole boneless, skinless chicken breasts

Instructions

1. In medium bowl, combine apples, chili pepper, onion, lime juice and salt and pepper to taste. Cover and set salsa aside while preparing chicken. You can refrigerate if making a day ahead of time.
2. In a large bowl, combine white wine, apple juice, lime zest, salt, and pepper. Cut chicken breasts in half for a total of four pieces. Add chicken and coat with mixture. Cover and refrigerate for at least half an hour.
3. Drain and discard chicken marinade.
4. Heat grill. Grill chicken until cooked through.
5. Serve with the salsa.

Curried Pork in Apple Cider
SERVINGS: 6

PREP TIME: **15 min.**
TOTAL TIME: **45 min.**

Ingredients

- 16 ounces pork tenderloin, cut into 6 pieces
- 1 1/2 tablespoons curry powder
- 1 tablespoon extra-virgin olive oil
- 2 medium yellow onions (about 2 cups), chopped
- 2 cups apple cider, divided
- 1 tart apple, peeled, seeded and chopped into chunks
- 1 tablespoon corn-starch

Instructions

1. Season pork tenderloin with curry powder. Let stand for 15 minutes.
2. Heat olive oil over medium-high heat in a large skillet. Add tenderloin and cook, turning once, until browned on both sides, around 5 to 10 minutes. Remove meat from skillet and set aside.
3. Add onions to skillet and sauté until golden and soft. Add 1 1/2 cups of the apple cider, reduce heat and simmer until the liquid is half gone.
4. Add chopped apple, corn-starch and remaining 1/2 cup apple cider. Simmer and stir while sauce thickens, about 2 minutes. Return tenderloin to skillet and simmer for the 5 minutes.
5. Pour thickened sauce over meat and serve immediately.

Halibut with Tomato and Basil Salsa
SERVINGS: 4

PREP TIME: **10 min.**
TOTAL TIME: **25 min.**

Ingredients

- 2 tomatoes, diced
- 2 tablespoons fresh basil, chopped
- 1 teaspoon fresh oregano, chopped
- 1 tablespoon minced garlic
- 2 teaspoons extra-virgin olive oil
- 4 halibut fillets, each 4 ounces

Instructions

1. Preheat oven to 350°F (175°C).
2. Lightly coat a 9-by-13-inch baking pan with cooking spray.
3. In a small bowl, combine tomato, basil, oregano and garlic. Add olive oil and mix well.
4. Arrange halibut fillets in the baking pan. Spoon tomato mixture on top of the fish.
5. Place in oven and bake until fish is opaque in the middle when tested with the tip of a knife, around 10 to 15 minutes.
6. Transfer individual plates and serve immediately.

Cranberry Chicken
SERVINGS: 4

PREP TIME: **5 min.**
TOTAL TIME: **20 min.**

Ingredients

- 1 pound boneless, skinless chicken breasts
- 1 teaspoon butter
- 1/4 teaspoon black pepper
- 3/4 cup whole cranberry sauce
- 1/4 cup chili sauce
- 1/4 cup apple juice
- 1 teaspoon brown sugar

Instructions

1. Sprinkle chicken with pepper. Pound the meat.
2. In a large pan, brown the chicken in butter.
3. Add remaining ingredients and simmer for 15 minutes, covered.
4. Remove lid and boil until sauce is desired thickness.

Whiskey-Mushroom New York Strip Steak
SERVINGS: 2

PREP TIME: **10 min.**
TOTAL TIME: **35 min.**

Ingredients

- 2 New York strip steaks (4 ounces each) trimmed of all visible fat
- 1 teaspoon margarine
- 3 garlic cloves, chopped
- 2 ounces sliced shiitake mushrooms
- 2 ounces button mushrooms
- 1/4 teaspoon thyme

- 1/4 teaspoon rosemary
- 1/4 cup whiskey

Instructions

1. Lightly coat grill rack or broiler pan with cooking spray and place cooking rack 4 to 6 inches from the heat source.
2. Preheat a gas grill or broiler.
3. Grill or broil the steaks, about 10 minutes on each side, until slightly pink on the inside, or until a food thermometer indicates 145°F (65°C), 160°F (70°C) (medium) or 170°F (75°C) (well done). Transfer to a plate and keep warm.
4. In a small saucepan, heat the margarine over medium heat. Add garlic, mushrooms, thyme and rosemary. Sauté until the mushrooms are tender, about 1 to 2 minutes. Remove and carefully add the whiskey (be careful of flame). Stir sauce for another minute.
5. Top steaks with mushrooms sauce and immediately serve.

Pear Curry Chicken
SERVINGS: 6

PREP TIME: **10 min.**
TOTAL TIME: **30 min.**

Ingredients

- 2 ripe pears, divided
- 1 tablespoon vegetable oil

- 1 cup diced onion
- 1 tablespoon curry powder
- 1 teaspoon minced garlic
- 1 teaspoon salt
- 3/4 teaspoon ground ginger
- 3/4 teaspoon ground cinnamon
- 1/4 teaspoon ground black pepper
- 3 chicken breasts (1 1/2 pounds), halved, boneless, skinless, cut into 1-inch cubes
- 1 can (14 ounces) light coconut milk
- 1/3 cup raisins (optional)

Instructions

1. Peel and core 1 pear. Puree and set aside.
2. Heat oil over medium heat in large frying pan. Add onion, curry powder, garlic, salt, ginger, cinnamon, and pepper and sauté 5 minutes, occasionally stirring, until onions are transparent.
3. Add chicken, and continue to sauté 5 minutes, stirring occasionally, until browned. A
4. Add pureed pear, coconut milk, and raisins. Simmer for 5 minutes.
5. Core and cut remaining pear into 1/2-inch cubes and add to curry. Simmer for 5 minutes and serve.

Mustard-Dill Poached Salmon
SERVINGS: 4

PREP TIME: **10 min.**
TOTAL TIME: **30 min.**

Ingredients

- 1 teaspoon olive or vegetable oil
- 2 tablespoon shallots, finely chopped
- 1 1/2 cup fat-free or low-fat milk
- 1/2 teaspoon salt
- Freshly ground black pepper to taste
- 1 1/4 pounds salmon fillet, about 1 inch thick, skin on, cut into 4 portions
- 1 tablespoons fresh lemon juice
- 1 1/2 teaspoons corn-starch
- 2 tablespoons chopped fresh dill
- 1/4 cup reduced-fat sour cream
- 2 teaspoons Dijon mustard
- Lemon wedges and fresh dill sprigs, for garnish

Instructions

1. Heat oil over medium heat in a large skillet or sauté pan. Add shallots and sauté until softened, about 30 to 60 seconds. Add milk, shallots, salt and pepper. Bring to simmer while stirring. Reduce heat to low.
2. Place salmon pieces in milk sauce, skin-side up, and immediately turn over. Cover and gently poach salmon, occasionally spooning milk liquid over top of salmon, about 10 to 12 minutes or just until interior is opaque.
3. Carefully transfer salmon to a warm platter. Cover with foil and keep warm.
4. In a small bowl, mix lemon juice and corn-starch. Add mix to poaching liquid and cook, constantly

stirring, until slightly thickened, about 1 minute. Stir in sour cream, chopped dill and mustard.
5. Garnish salmon with lemon wedges and dill sprigs. Serve with the mustard-dill sauce.

Fish Cod Fillet Tacos
SERVINGS: 8

PREP TIME: **15 min.**
TOTAL TIME: **35 min.**

Ingredients
Fish

- 2 pounds cod fillets
- 3 tablespoons lime juice (or juice from 2 limes)
- 1 tomato, chopped
- 1/2 onion, chopped
- 3 tablespoons cilantro, chopped
- 1 teaspoon olive oil
- 1/4 teaspoon cayenne pepper (optional)
- 1/4 teaspoon black pepper
- 1/4 teaspoon salt

Slaw

- 2 cups red cabbage, shredded
- 1/2 cup green onions, chopped
- 3/4 cup non-fat sour cream
- 3/4 cup salsa
- 8 6-inch corn tortillas

Instructions

1. Preheat oven to 350°F (175°C).
2. Rinse fish and drain fat off by placing on rack in baking dish.
3. Combine lime juice, tomato, onion, cilantro, olive oil, peppers, and salt and spoon on top of fillets. Keep fish moist by covering loosely with aluminium foil. Bake 15-20 minutes or until fish flakes.
4. Mix cabbage and onion.
5. Combine sour cream and salsa and add to cabbage mixture.
6. Divide fish among tortillas. Add 1/4 cup of slaw to each.

Garlic and Lime Pork Chops
SERVINGS: 4

PREP TIME: **20 min.**
TOTAL TIME: **35 min.**

Ingredients

- 4 (6 ounces each) lean boneless pork chops
- 4 cloves garlic, crushed
- 1 teaspoon cumin
- 1 teaspoon chili powder
- 1 teaspoon paprika
- Fresh black pepper to taste
- 1 tablespoon of lime juice (about 1/2 lime)
- Zest of 1/2 lime (about 1 teaspoon)

Instructions

1. Trim fat off pork.
2. In a large bowl season pork with garlic, cumin, chili powder, paprika, and pepper. Add lime juice and lime zest. Allow pork to marinate for at least 20 minutes.
3. Line a broiler pan with foil. Place pork chops on the broiler pan and broil for around 4-5 minutes on each side, or until browned.

Honey Crusted Chicken
SERVINGS: 2

PREP TIME: **10 min.**
TOTAL TIME: **35 min.**

Ingredients

- 8 saltine crackers, each about 2 inches
- 1 teaspoon paprika
- 2 boneless, skinless chicken breasts (4 ounces each)
- 4 teaspoons honey

Instructions

1. Preheat oven to 375°F (190°C). Lightly coat baking dish with cooking spray.
2. Crush crackers and place in a small bowl. Add paprika and mix well.
3. Add chicken and honey in a separate bowl. Toss to evenly coat. Add cracker mixture and press chicken in until it's evenly coated on both sides.

4. Place chicken in the prepared baking dish. Bake until lightly browned and cooked through, about 20 to 25 minutes. Serve immediately.

Spicy Mango Jerk Chicken
SERVINGS: 4

PREP TIME: **20 min**
TOTAL TIME: **45 min**

Ingredients

- 2 ripe mangos, peeled, pitted and cut into 1/4-inches
- 1/4 cup lime juice
- 2 tablespoon brown sugar
- 1/2 teaspoon crushed red pepper
- 1/4 teaspoon garlic powder
- 1/4 teaspoon cinnamon
- 1/4 teaspoon ground allspice
- 4 boneless, skinless chicken breasts, slightly flattened (about 1 1/2 pounds)
- 2 tablespoon Jamaican jerk seasoning blend
- 1 lime, halved

Instructions

1. In a medium bowl, combine mango, lime juice, brown sugar, red pepper, garlic powder, cinnamon and allspice. Set aside.
2. Rinse chicken and pat dry. Sprinkle both sides with jerk seasoning and let stand for 10 minutes.

3. Cook on a well-oiled grill over medium heat for about 5 to 7 minutes on each side, or until chicken is cooked through. Remove and squeeze lime halves over chicken.
4. Top with spicy mango mixture.

Lemon Chicken and Potatoes
SERVINGS: 4

PREP TIME: **10 min.**
TOTAL TIME: **45 min.**

Ingredients

- 1 1/2 pounds boneless skinless chicken breasts, cut into 1-inch cubes
- 1 pound Yukon Gold potatoes, cut into 3/4-inch cubes
- 1 medium onion, coarsely chopped
- 1/2 cup reduced-fat Greek or olive oil vinaigrette
- 1/4 cup lemon juice
- 1 teaspoon dry oregano
- 1 teaspoon minced garlic
- 1/2 cup chopped tomato

Instructions

1. In a large bowl, mix all ingredients except tomatoes. Place equal amounts on 4 large squares of heavy-duty aluminium foil. Enclose and fold sides of each to enclose filling. Leave room to allow air to circulate.

2. Grill over medium heat for 25 to 30 minutes or until chicken is cooked through and potatoes are soft.
3. Carefully open each foil and sprinkle equal amounts of tomato.

Pork Medallions with Herbes de Provence
SERVINGS: 2

PREP TIME: **10 min.**
TOTAL TIME: **25 min.**

Ingredients

- 8 ounces pork tenderloin, trimmed of visible fat and cut crosswise into 6 pieces
- Freshly ground black pepper, to taste
- 1/2 teaspoon herbes de Provence
- 1/4 cup dry white wine

Instructions

1. Sprinkle pork with black pepper. Place pork between sheets of wax paper and pound with a mallet or roll with a rolling pin until about 1/4-inch thick.
2. In a large, non-stick frying pan, cook the pork over medium-high heat, about 2 to 3 minutes on each side. Remove from heat and sprinkle with herbes de Provence. Place the pork on individual plates and keep warm.
3. Pour wine into frying pan and cook until boiling. Scrape brown bits from the bottom of the pan. Pour

the wine sauce over the pork and serve immediately.

Pork Tenderloin with Apples and Balsamic Vinegar

SERVINGS: 4

PREP TIME: **10 min.**
TOTAL TIME: **35 min.**

Ingredients

- 1 tablespoon olive oil
- 1 pound pork tenderloin, trimmed of all visible fat
- Freshly ground black pepper, to taste
- 2 cups chopped onion
- 2 cups chopped apple
- 1 1/2 tablespoons fresh rosemary, chopped
- 1 cup low-sodium chicken broth
- 1 1/2 tablespoons balsamic vinegar

Instructions

1. Preheat oven to 450°F (230°C). Lightly coat a baking pan with cooking spray.
2. In a large skillet, heat olive oil over high heat. Add pork and sprinkle with black pepper. Cook until browned on all sides, about 3 minutes. Remove from heat and place in the prepared baking pan. Roast the pork for 15 minutes, or until a food thermometer reads 165°F (75°C) (medium).

3. Add onion, apple and rosemary to the skillet. Sauté over medium heat, about 3 to 5 minutes or until onions and apples are soft. Stir in the broth and vinegar. Increase heat and boil until the sauce is reduced, about 5 minutes.
4. Place pork on a large platter. Slice on the diagonal and put on 4 warmed plates. Scoop onion-apple sauce over top and serve immediately.

Salsa Verde Burger
SERVINGS: 4

PREP TIME: **15 min.**
TOTAL TIME: **45 min.**

Ingredients
- 2 tomatillos
- 1 serrano chile pepper, sliced
- 1/4 cup onion, sliced
- 1/4 teaspoon chopped garlic
- 1 teaspoon black pepper
- 4 (93% lean) beef patties (4.75 ounces each)
- 1/2 cup salsa verde
- 4 slices reduced-fat pepper jack cheese
- 4 whole-wheat hamburger buns
- 1/4 cup shredded red cabbage
- 4 ounces sliced avocado

Instructions

1. Place the tomatillos, Serrano peppers, onion, and garlic in a saucepan. Just cover with water and bring to a boil. Reduce heat to medium-low and cook until the tomatillos are soft and are slightly brown, about 20-30 minutes. Add more water if needed to keep from burning.
2. Pour cooked vegetables into a blender and blend until smooth.
3. Heat a skillet or grill over high heat.
4. When hot, spray with cooking spray or lightly oil. Add the patties.
5. Season with pepper and cook a few minutes on each side, as desired.
6. Add cheese and cover. Cook to melt, about 30 seconds.
7. Place the cooked burgers on the buns and top each with 2 tablespoons salsa verde, red cabbage, and avocado slices.

Brazilian Black Beans Sausage
SERVINGS: 8

PREP TIME: **15 min.**
TOTAL TIME: **50 min.**

Ingredients

- 2 teaspoons vegetable oil
- 8 ounces low-fat polish kielbasa sausage, cut into small pieces
- 1 large onion, chopped

- 1/8 teaspoon garlic powder or 1 clove garlic, minced
- 1 red bell pepper, chopped
- 1 teaspoon ground cumin
- 1 cup brown uncooked rice
- 1 can (15 ounces) black beans, drained and rinsed
- 2 cups water
- Mushrooms and/or bell peppers, optional
- Cayenne pepper, if desired

Instructions

1. Heat oil over medium-high heat and sauté sausage and onion until onion becomes translucent.
2. Add the remaining ingredients and bring to boil over high heat. Reduce heat to low, cover and simmer for 40 minutes.

Tangy Yogurt Broiled Halibut
SERVINGS: 2

PREP TIME: **10 min.**
TOTAL TIME: **20 min.**

Ingredients
- 2 halibut fillets (5 ounces each)
- 1 cup non-fat plain yogurt
- 1 large clove garlic, peeled and crushed
- 1/4 teaspoon ground black pepper
- 1/4 cup freshly squeezed lemon juice
- 1/4 teaspoon salt

Instructions

1. Preheat broiler.
2. In a small bowl, combine yogurt, lemon juice, garlic, salt and pepper. Mix well.
3. Line a broiler pan with foil and place fish on top with the skin side down. Spread half of yogurt sauce over fish. Place fish 4 inches under broiler and cook for 10 minutes, or until fish flakes easily with a fork and topping is golden.
4. Serve warm with the rest of the yogurt sauce on the side.

Mediterranean-Style Grilled Salmon
SERVINGS: 4

PREP TIME: **10 min.**
TOTAL TIME: **25 min.**

Ingredients

- 4 tablespoons chopped fresh basil
- 1 tablespoon chopped fresh parsley
- 1 tablespoon minced garlic
- 2 tablespoons lemon juice
- 4 salmon fillets (5 ounces each)
- Black pepper, to taste
- 4 green olives, chopped
- 4 thin slices lemon

Instructions

1. Lightly coat grill rack or broiler pan with cooking spray and place cooking rack 4 to 6 inches from the heat source.
2. Preheat a gas grill or broiler.
3. Combine basil, parsley, minced garlic and lemon juice in a small bowl.
4. Spray fillets with cooking spray and sprinkle with black pepper. Top each with equal amounts of the basil-garlic mixture.
5. Place fillets herb-side down on grill over high heat. When edges turn white, turn fillets over and place on aluminium foil, about 3 to 4 minutes. Move to a cooler part of grill or reduce the heat. Grill until the opaque throughout when tested with the tip of a knife, about 4 more minutes.
6. Remove salmon and place on warmed plates. Garnish with green olives and lemon slices.

Chicken with Oranges and Avocados
SERVINGS: 4
PREP/TOTAL TIME: 35 min. + refrigeration

Ingredients
- 1 cup low-fat yogurt
- 1/4 cup minced red onion
- 1 tablespoon honey
- salt and ground black pepper, to taste
- 4 boneless skinless chicken breasts (4-6 ounce each)

Garnish

- 1 avocado
- 1/4 cup fresh lime juice
- 2 oranges, peeled and sectioned
- 2 tablespoon chopped cilantro
- 1 small red onion, thinly sliced

Instructions

1. In a large bowl, combine all the ingredients except the chicken and garnish. Add chicken to the mix and coat evenly. Cover and refrigerate for half an hour.
2. Preheat the grill or broiler.
3. Remove the chicken from the marinade. Sprinkle with salt and pepper.
4. Place chicken on the grill or under the broiler. Cook until juices run clear.
5. While the chicken is cooking, peel, core and chop the avocado and combine it with the lime juice quickly. Add oranges, onion and cilantro.
6. Season with salt and serve on top of chicken.

Lime and Cilantro Tilapia Tacos
SERVINGS: 2

PREP TIME: **10 min.**
TOTAL TIME: **35 min.**

Ingredients

- 1 pound tilapia filets, rinsed and patted dry
- 1 teaspoon olive oil
- 1 small onion, chopped

- 4 cloves garlic, finely minced
- 2 jalapeno peppers, chopped, and seeds removed
- 2 cups diced tomatoes
- 1/4 cup fresh cilantro, chopped
- 3 tablespoons lime juice
- Salt and pepper, to taste
- 8 5-inch white corn tortillas
- 1 medium avocado, sliced into 8 slices
- 1 cup shredded cabbage
- Lime wedges and fresh chopped cilantro, for garnish
- 4 tablespoons low-fat or fat free sour cream, optional

Instructions

1. Heat olive oil in a skillet. Sauté onion until translucent. Add garlic and mix well.
2. Place tilapia in skillet and cook until the flesh begins to flake.
3. Add jalapeno peppers, tomatoes, cilantro and lime juice.
4. Sauté over medium-high heat for about 5 minutes, breaking up the fish and mixing well.
5. Season to taste with salt and pepper.
6. Heat tortillas on a skillet on each side to warm for a few minutes.
7. Serve 1/4 cup of fish on each warmed tortilla with two avocado slices.
8. Split 1/4 cup of shredded cabbage and 1 tablespoon of low-fat or fat free sour cream between 2 tacos, if using.

9. Garnish with fresh chopped cilantro and lime wedges.

Sesame Baked Chicken Tenders
SERVINGS: 4

PREP TIME: **10 min.**
TOTAL TIME: **25 min.**

Ingredients
- 16 ounces chicken tenderloins
- 2 teaspoons sesame oil
- 2 teaspoons low sodium soy sauce
- 6 tablespoons toasted sesame seeds
- 1/2 teaspoon coarse salt
- 4 tablespoons breadcrumbs (no salt added)
- olive oil spray

Instructions
1. Preheat oven to 425°F (220°C). Spray a baking sheet with non-stick oil spray or parchment paper.
2. In a bowl, combine sesame oil and soy sauce.
3. In a separate bowl, combine sesame seeds, salt, and panko.
4. Place chicken in with the oil and soy sauce, and then place into sesame seed mix to coat well.
5. Place on baking sheet and lightly spray top of the chicken with oil spray. Bake 8-10 minutes. Turn and cook another 5 minutes or until cooked through.

Spicy Pork with Sweet Potatoes and Apples
SERVINGS: 4

PREP TIME: **15 min.**
TOTAL TIME: **55 min.**

Ingredients

- 3/4 cup apple cider
- 1/4 cup apple cider vinegar
- 2 tablespoons maple syrup
- 1/4 teaspoon smoked paprika
- 1 teaspoon grated fresh ginger or 1/4 teaspoon dried ginger
- 1 teaspoon ground black pepper
- 2 teaspoons vegetable oil
- 1 (12 ounce) pork tenderloin
- 1 large sweet potato, cut into 1/4 to 1/2-inch cubes
- 1 large apple, cut into 1/2 inch cubes

Instructions

1. Preheat oven to 375°F (190°C).
2. In a medium bowl, combine apple cider, apple cider vinegar, maple syrup, smoked paprika, ginger, and black pepper. Set aside.
3. Heat oil over medium-high heat in a large ovenproof sauté pan with a lid. Once oil starts to smoke, reduce heat to medium and gently place pork in pan. Cook, and turn until all sides are well browned, about 8 to 12 minutes. Remove pan from heat.
4. Place sweet potatoes around pork and pour apple cider mix over the tenderloin. Cover and bake for 20

minutes. Roast until instant-read thermometer inserted into the thickest part of the tenderloin reads 145–150°F (65°C).

5. Turn sweet potatoes and place apple quarters around pork. Bake uncovered for another 5 to 10 minutes, or until tenderloin registers 170°F (75°C). Remove pork, apples, and sweet potatoes from roasting pan. Let pork stand for 10 minutes before slicing.

6. As pork is resting, reduce cider mix to about a 1/4 cup. Slice roasted pork into 1/2 thick pieces. Serve with the sweet potatoes and apples and pour reduced cider over everything on the plate.

Glazed Turkey Breast with Fruit Stuffing
SERVINGS: 12

PREP TIME: **15 min.**
TOTAL TIME: **2 1/2 hours**

Ingredients

- 1-5 pound whole, bone-in turkey breast, thawed

  Rub:

- 2 tablespoons fresh rosemary, chopped
- 2 tablespoons fresh thyme leaves, chopped
- 2 tablespoons olive oil

  Stuffing:

- 1 small onion, thinly sliced
- 1 apple, peeled and thinly sliced

93

- 1 pear, peeled and thinly sliced
- 1/4 cup dried cranberries (or raisins)

   Glaze:

- 2 cups (divided) apple juice
- 1 tablespoon brown sugar
- 1 tablespoon brown mustard
- 1 tablespoon olive oil

Instructions

1. Preheat oven to 325°F (165°C). Place turkey breast in a roasting pan, skin side up, on a rack.
2. In a small bowl, make a paste by combining the herbs and the olive oil. Loosen the skin from the meat with your fingers by making two deep pockets between skin and meat. Smear half the paste on the meat. Spread paste evenly over the top of the skin.
3. In another small bowl, mix the sliced onions and fruit. Stuff each pocket with the mixture.
4. Pour 1 cup of apple juice into the bottom of the roasting pan. Roast turkey breast for 1 hour 45 minutes to 2 hours, or until the skin is golden brown and a thermometer reads 165°F (73°C) when inserted into the thickest areas of the breast. If skin over-browns, cover breast loosely with aluminium foil.
5. In a sauce pan, combine remaining cup of apple juice, brown sugar, mustard and olive oil. Heat to boil. Reduce heat and simmer until it has thickened and reduced in volume to about 3/4 cup. Use to

baste the turkey during the last half hour of cooking.
6. When turkey is done, cover with foil and allow to rest at room temperature for 15 minutes.
7. Carve, serve and spoon remaining glaze over the turkey.

Pork Chops with Black Currant Sauce
SERVINGS: 6

PREP TIME: **10 min.**
TOTAL TIME: **30 min.**

Ingredients

- 1/4 cup black currant jam
- 2 tablespoons Dijon mustard
- 2 teaspoons olive oil
- 6 center cut pork loin chops (4 ounces each), trimmed of all visible fat
- 1/3 cup wine vinegar
- 1/8 teaspoon freshly ground black pepper
- 6 orange slices

Instructions

1. In a small bowl, whisk together jam and mustard.
2. In a large non-stick frying pan, heat olive oil over medium-high heat. Add pork chops and cook, until browned on both sides, about 5 minutes on each side. Top each pork chop with 1 tablespoon of the

jam-mustard mix. Cover and cook for 2 more minutes. Transfer to warmed plates.
3. Cool frying pan to a warm, but not hot, temperature. Pour wine vinegar into pan and stir to remove the bits of pork and jam. Pour vinegar sauce over each pork chop. Sprinkle with pepper and garnish with orange slices.
4. Serve immediately.

Honey Mustard Grilled Chicken with Toasted Almonds

SERVINGS: 4

PREP TIME: **10 min.**
TOTAL TIME: **30 min.**

Ingredients
- 1/4 cup Dijon mustard
- 3 teaspoon honey
- 1 teaspoon lemon juice
- 1 clove garlic, crushed
- 4 boneless, skinless chicken breasts
- 1/4 cup sliced almonds, toasted

Instructions
1. Preheat grill or broiler.
2. In a small bowl, combine mustard, honey, lemon juice, and garlic.
3. Brush chicken with the honey mustard sauce on both sides.

96

4. Grill or broil 6 inches from heat source for 10-15 minutes, occasionally turning and brushing with additional sauce; except for last 5 minutes. Discard remaining honey mustard sauce.
5. Sprinkle with almonds and serve.

Grilled Pesto Shrimp Skewers
SERVINGS: 7

PREP TIME: **20 min.**

> **TOTAL TIME:** 30 min. + refrigeration

Ingredients

- 1 cup fresh basil leaves, chopped
- 1 clove garlic, peeled
- 1/4 cup grated Parmigiano Reggiano cheese
- 3 tablespoons olive oil
- 1 1/2 pounds (weight after peeling) jumbo shrimp, peeled and deveined
- Salt and pepper, to taste
- 7 wooden skewers

Instructions

1. Pulse basil, garlic, parmesan cheese, salt and pepper in a food processor until smooth. Slowly add oil during pulsing. In a bowl, combine raw shrimp with pesto. Cover and marinate in the refrigerator for a few hours.

2. Soak wooden skewers in water for at least 20 minutes (or just use metal ones). Place the shrimp on skewers

3. Heat a grill pan over medium-low heat. Spray lightly with olive oil. Place shrimp on the grill and cook until they are pink on the bottom, about 3-4 minutes. Turn and cook until shrimp is opaque and cooked, about 3-4 more minutes.

Grilled Pork Fajitas
SERVINGS: 8

PREP TIME: **10 min.**
TOTAL TIME: **25 min.**

Ingredients
- 1 tablespoon chili powder
- 1/2 teaspoon oregano
- 1/2 teaspoon paprika
- 1/4 teaspoon ground coriander
- 1/4 teaspoon garlic powder
- 1 pound pork tenderloin, cut into strips 1/2 inch wide and 2 inches long
- 1 small onion, sliced
- 8 whole-wheat flour tortillas, about 8 inches in diameter, warmed in microwave
- 1/2 cup shredded sharp cheddar cheese
- 4 medium tomatoes, diced
- 4 cups shredded lettuce
- 1 cup salsa

Instructions

1. Heat a gas grill or broiler to medium-high heat or 400°F (200°C).
2. In a small bowl, combine and stir the chili powder, oregano, paprika, coriander and garlic powder. Coat the pork pieces completely in the seasonings.
3. In a cast-iron pan or grill basket, place the pork strips and onions. Grill or broil at medium-high heat until browned on all sides, about 5 minutes, turning several times.
4. Spread an equal amount of pork strips and onions on each tortilla. Top each with 1 tablespoon cheese, 2 tablespoons tomatoes, 1/2 cup shredded lettuce and 2 tablespoons salsa.
5. Fold in both sides of each tortilla, and roll to close.
6. Serve immediately.

Southeast Asian Baked Salmon

SERVINGS: **2**

PREP TIME: **10 min.**

TOTAL TIME: 35 min. + marinating

Ingredients

- 1/2 cup pineapple juice, no sugar added
- 2 garlic cloves, minced
- 1 teaspoon low-sodium soy sauce
- 1/4 teaspoon ground ginger
- 2 salmon fillets, 4 ounces each
- 1/4 teaspoon sesame oil

- Freshly ground black pepper, to taste
- 1 cup diced fresh fruit, such as pineapple, mango and papaya

Instructions

1. Add pineapple juice, garlic, soy sauce and ginger in a small bowl. Stir and evenly combine. In a small baking dish, arrange salmon fillets. Pour pineapple juice mix on top. Place in refrigerator and marinate for an hour. Turn the salmon occasionally as needed.
2. Heat oven to 375°F (190°C).
3. Lightly coat two squares of aluminium foil with cooking spray. Place marinated salmon fillets on aluminium foil. Drizzle each fillet with 1/8 teaspoon sesame oil. Sprinkle with pepper and top with 1/2 cup diced fruit on each. Wrap foil around the salmon and fold to seal edges. Bake about 10 minutes on each side, until fish is opaque throughout when cut with a knife.
4. Transfer salmon to individual plates and immediately serve.

Grilled Snapper Curry
SERVINGS: 4

PREP TIME: **10 min.**
TOTAL TIME: **25 min.**

Ingredients

- 1/2 teaspoon coconut extract

- 1 teaspoon black pepper
- 1/2 teaspoon fennel seed
- 1 tablespoon turmeric
- 1 teaspoon coriander
- 1 teaspoon cumin
- 1 teaspoon paprika
- 1 cup soy or skim milk
- 1 teaspoon corn-starch
- 1 teaspoon canola oil
- 2 tablespoons fresh ginger, minced
- 1 poblano pepper, sliced
- 2 cups sliced bok choy
- 2 cups sliced celery
- 1 cup sliced red bell pepper
- 1 cup sliced onion
- 2 cloves garlic, minced
- 4 six-ounce red snapper fillets

Instructions

1. Mix coconut extract and spices with milk and corn-starch. Set aside.
2. Place large skillet on medium-high heat. Add oil and sauté vegetables for a few minutes, until browned and vegetables are soft. Add milk and spice mixture to pan and stir. Heat gently, but do not boil. Remove from heat.
3. Broil or grill snapper until cooked or it reaches a temperature of 145°F (65°C).
4. Serve each fillet with 1 1/2 cups of vegetables and sauce.

Roasted Salmon with Maple Glaze
SERVINGS: 6

PREP TIME: **10 min.**
TOTAL TIME: **45 min.**

Ingredients

- 1/4 cup maple syrup
- 1 garlic clove, minced
- 1/4 cup balsamic vinegar
- 2 pounds salmon, cut into 6 equal-sized fillets
- 1/4 teaspoon kosher or sea salt
- 1/8 teaspoon fresh cracked black pepper
- Fresh mint or parsley for garnish

Instructions

1. Preheat oven to 450°F (230°C). Lightly coat a baking pan with cooking spray.
2. Mix together the maple syrup, garlic and balsamic vinegar in a small saucepan over low heat. Heat until hot and then remove from heat. Pour half of mix into a small bowl for basting, and reserve the rest for later.
3. Pat salmon dry. Place skin-side down on baking sheet. Brush salmon with the maple syrup mix. Bake about 10 minutes, and brush again with maple syrup mix, and bake for 5 more minutes. Continue to baste and bake until fish flakes easily, about 20 to 25 minutes in total.
4. Transfer salmon to plates.

5. Sprinkle with salt and black pepper, and top with reserved maple syrup mix. Garnish with fresh mint or parsley and serve immediately.

Spinach, Shrimp and Feta with Tuscan White Beans

SERVINGS: 4

PREP TIME: **5 min.**
TOTAL TIME: **15 min.**

Ingredients

- 2 tablespoons olive oil
- 1 pound large shrimp, peeled and deveined
- 1 medium onion, chopped
- 4 cloves garlic, minced
- 2 teaspoons chopped fresh sage
- 2 tablespoons balsamic vinegar
- 1/2 cup low sodium, fat-free chicken broth
- 15 ounce can no-salt added cannellini beans, rinsed and drained
- 5 cups baby spinach
- 1 1/2 ounce crumbled reduced-fat feta cheese

Instructions

1. In a large non-stick skillet, heat 1 teaspoon oil over medium-high heat. Cook shrimp until opaque, about 2 to 3 minutes. Transfer to a plate.
2. Heat remaining oil over medium-high heat and add onion, garlic and sage. Cook for 4 minutes

occasionally stirring until golden. Stir in vinegar and cook 30 seconds.

3. Add broth, bring to a boil and cook 2 minutes. Stir in beans and spinach and cook about 2 to 3 minutes, until the spinach wilts. Remove from heat and stir in shrimp.
4. Top with feta cheese and divide in 4 bowls.

DESSERTS

Red, White, and Blue Fruit Skewers and Cheesecake Dip

SERVINGS: **24**
PREP/TOTAL TIME: **20 min.**

Ingredients

Cheesecake dipping sauce:

- 4 ounces 1/3 less fat cream cheese, softened
- 1 cup fat free Greek yogurt
- 1 teaspoon vanilla extract
- 1/4 cup sugar

Skewers:

- 14 ounces angel food cake, cut into 1-inch cubes
- 72-84 medium strawberries (about 3 1/2 pounds), stems removed
- 1 pint blueberries

- 24-28 skewers

Instructions

1. Combine cream cheese with yogurt, vanilla and sugar in a medium bowl. Mix until sugar dissolves and set aside.
2. Thread 3 strawberries and 2 cubes of cake onto each skewer. Alternate between strawberries and cake. Finish each skewer with 3 blueberries and place finished skewers on a platter.
3. Refrigerate skewers and dip until ready to serve.

Honey and Yogurt Grilled Peaches

SERVINGS: **4**
PREP TIME: **5 min.**
TOTAL TIME: **10 min.**

Ingredients

- 2 large ripe peaches, cut in half (pit removed)
- 1/4 cup fat free vanilla Greek yogurt
- 1/8 teaspoon cinnamon
- 2 tablespoons honey

Instructions

1. Heat grill to low heat.
2. Grill peaches, covered on low or indirect heat about 2-4 minutes on each side or until soft.
3. In a small bowl combine yogurt and cinnamon.
4. When the peaches are cooked, drizzle with honey and top each with 1 tablespoon of yogurt.

Blackberry Cinnamon Ginger Iced Tea

SERVINGS: **7**
PREP TIME: **5 min.**
TOTAL TIME: **20 min.**

Ingredients

- 6 cups water
- 12 blackberry herbal tea bags
- 8 cinnamon sticks (3-inch-long)
- 1 tablespoon minced fresh ginger
- 1 cup unsweetened cranberry juice
- Sugar, to taste
- Ice cubes, crushed

Instructions

1. Heat water in a large saucepan, but avoid boiling. Add tea bags, two cinnamon sticks and ginger. Remove from heat, cover and steep for about 15 minutes.
2. Pass mix through a sieve into a pitcher. Add juice and sweetener to taste. Refrigerate until cold.
3. To serve, fill six tall glasses with crushed ice. Pour tea over the top of ice and garnish with cinnamon sticks.
4. Serve immediately.

Apples and Cream Shake

SERVINGS: **4**

PREP/TOTAL TIME: **5 min.**

Ingredients
- 2 cups vanilla low-fat ice cream
- 1 cup unsweetened applesauce
- 1/4 teaspoon ground cinnamon or apple pie spice
- 1 cup fat-free skim milk

Instructions.
1. In a blender, combine low-fat ice cream, applesauce and cinnamon or apple pie spice. Cover and blend until smooth.
2. Add fat-free skim milk. Cover and blend until well-mixed.
3. Pour into glasses. Sprinkle each serving with an additional cinnamon, if desired.
4. Serve immediately.

Fruited Rice Pudding
SERVINGS: **8**
PREP TIME: **10 min.**
TOTAL TIME: 1 hour 15 min.

Ingredients
- 2 cups water
- 1 cup long-grain rice
- 4 cups evaporated fat-free milk
- 1/2 cup brown sugar

- 1/2 teaspoon lemon zest
- 1 teaspoon vanilla extract
- 6 egg whites
- 1/4 cup crushed pineapple
- 1/4 cup raisins
- 1/4 cup chopped apricots

Instructions

1. Bring 2 cups of water to a boil in a medium saucepan. Add rice and cook for about 10 minutes. Pour into a colander and thoroughly drain.
2. In the same saucepan, add the evaporated milk and brown sugar, cooking until hot. Add the cooked rice, lemon zest and vanilla extract. Simmer over low heat until the mix is thick and rice is tender, about 30 minutes Remove from the heat and cool down.
3. In a small bowl whisk the egg whites together. Pour into the rice mix. Add pineapple, raisins and apricots. Stir until blended.
4. Preheat oven to 325°F (165°C). Lightly coat a baking dish with cooking spray.
5. Spoon pudding and fruit mix into the baking dish. Bake until the pudding is set, about 20 minutes.
6. Serve warm or cold.

SNACKS AND SIDES

Sweet and Spicy Roasted Red Pepper Hummus

SERVINGS: **8**

PREP/TOTAL TIME: **10 min.**

Ingredients

- 1 (15 ounce) can garbanzo (chickpeas) beans, drained
- 1 (4 ounce) jar roasted red peppers
- 3 tablespoons lemon juice
- 1 1/2 tablespoons tahini
- 1 clove garlic, minced
- 1/2 teaspoon ground cumin
- 1/2 teaspoon cayenne pepper
- 1/4 teaspoon salt
- 1 tablespoon chopped fresh parsley

Instructions

1. Puree chickpeas, red peppers, lemon juice, tahini, garlic, cumin, cayenne, and salt in an electric blender or food processor. Process using long pulses until smooth and slightly fluffy. Scrape the mixture off the sides between pulses. Transfer to a serving bowl and refrigerate at least an hour.
2. Return to room temperature before serving. Sprinkle with the chopped parsley before serving.

Chipotle Spiced Shrimp

SERVINGS: 4

PREP TIME:

TOTAL TIME:

Ingredients

- 3/4 pound uncooked shrimp, peeled and deveined (about 48 shrimps)
- 2 tablespoons tomato paste
- 1 1/2 teaspoons water
- 1/2 teaspoon extra-virgin olive oil
- 1/2 teaspoon minced garlic
- 1/2 teaspoon chipotle chili powder
- 1/2 teaspoon fresh oregano, chopped

Instructions

1. Rinse shrimp in cold water and pat dry with a paper towel. Set aside.
2. In a small bowl whisk together tomato paste, water and oil. Mix in garlic, chili powder and oregano.
3. Using a brush, spread the marinade mix on both sides of the shrimp. Place in the refrigerator.
4. Preheat a gas grill or broiler. Lightly coat grill rack or broiler pan with cooking spray. Position the cooking rack 4 to 6 inches from the heat source.
5. Put shrimp in grill basket or on skewers and place on the grill. Turn shrimp after 3 to 4 minutes.

Lemon Glaze
SERVINGS: 4
PREP/ TOTAL TIME: **5 min.**

Ingredients

- 1 teaspoon lemon or lime juice
- 1 teaspoon grated lemon or lime zest
- 1/2 cup unsalted chicken broth
- 1 tablespoon chopped parsley
- 1 tablespoon sugar
- 2 teaspoons corn-starch

Instructions

1. Combine all the ingredients in a microwavable bowl. Whisk and mix evenly. Microwave on high until clear and thickened, about 1 to 2 minutes.
2. Serve immediately with chicken, fish, or vegetables.

Maple Mustard Kale with Turkey Bacon

SERVINGS: 4

PREP TIME: **5 min.**
TOTAL TIME: **10 min.**

Ingredients

- 1 tsp olive oil
- 1/2 large onion, sliced
- 3 strips turkey bacon cut crosswise into strips
- 1 bunch kale
- 1 tablespoon whole grained mustard
- 1 teaspoon apple cider vinegar
- 1 tablespoon 100% pure maple syrup

Instructions

1. Remove tough ribs from kale. Cut into bite-size pieces. Wash well and pat dry.
2. Heat a large sauté pan over medium heat. Add olive oil, onions and turkey bacon and sauté about 8 minutes or until browned.
3. Add washed kale and cook until wilted, stirring occasionally, for about 4 minutes.
4. Combine whole grain mustard, apple cider vinegar and pure maple syrup, in a small bowl.
5. When kale is wilted and tender, drizzle mustard mix over the kale and stir to combine. Heat for about 1 minute. Serve warm.

Garlic and Kale with Black-Eyed Peas

SERVINGS: **6**
PREP TIME: **10 min.**
TOTAL TIME: **30 min.**

Ingredients

- 1 1/2 pounds kale, washed and drained
- 1 teaspoon olive or other vegetable oil
- 1 teaspoon chopped fresh garlic, or more to taste
- Pinch of dried red pepper flakes
- 2 cup canned black-eyed peas, drained (or cooked from dry)
- 1 teaspoon cider vinegar, to taste

Instructions

1. Pull kale leaves from tough stems. Discard stems and chop leaves into one-inch pieces.
2. Place two inches of water in a large pot and boil. Add kale, cover and cook 15 to 20 minutes or until tender, stirring occasionally. Drain, reserving water for soup if desired.
3. Heat a large non-stick skillet over medium-low heat. Add oil and garlic. Cook garlic while stirring, about 2 minutes or until it begins to sizzle.
4. Add black-eyed peas and red pepper flakes and cook about 3 minutes or until heated through, stirring occasionally.
5. Add kale and stir to combine over low heat.
6. Add cider vinegar just before serving.

Sweet and Spicy Snack Mix

SERVINGS: **4**
PREP TIME: **5 min.**
TOTAL TIME: **50 min.**

Ingredients

- butter-flavored cooking spray
- 2 cans (15 ounces each) garbanzos beans (chickpeas), rinsed, drained and patted dry
- 2 cups wheat squares cereal
- 1 cup dried pineapple chunks
- 1 cup raisins
- 2 tablespoons honey
- 2 tablespoons Worcestershire sauce

- 1 teaspoon garlic powder
- 1/2 teaspoon chili powder

Instructions

1. Preheat oven to 350°F (175°C). Lightly coat a 15 1/2-inch-by-10 1/2-inch baking sheet with butter-flavored cooking spray or grease.
2. Spray a heavy skillet generously with butter-flavored cooking spray. Add garbanzos and cook over medium heat. Stir frequently for about 10 minutes or until beans begin to brown. Transfer to the prepared baking sheet. Spray beans lightly with cooking spray. Bake about 20 minutes, stirring frequently until beans are crisp.
3. Lightly coat a roasting pan with butter-flavored cooking spray. Add cereal, pineapple, raisins and roasted garbanzos to pan. Stir to evenly mix.
4. In a large measuring cup combine honey, Worcestershire sauce and spices. Stir to evenly mix. Pour over the snack mix and gently toss. Spray mix again with cooking spray. Bake for 10 to 15 minutes, stirring occasionally to keep from burning.
5. Remove from oven and let cool.

Baked Pears with Walnuts and Honey

SERVINGS: **4**
PREP TIME: **15 min.**
TOTAL TIME: **45 min.**

Ingredients

- 2 large ripe pears
- 1/4 teaspoon ground cinnamon
- 2 teaspoon honey
- 1/4 cup crushed walnuts

Instructions

1. Preheat the oven to 350°F (175°C).
2. Cut pears in half and place on a baking sheet and scoop out the seeds.
3. Sprinkle with cinnamon. Top with walnuts and drizzle 1/2 teaspoon honey over each one.
4. Bake in the oven 30 minutes.
5. Let cool and serve.

Classic Boston Baked Beans

SERVINGS: **12**
PREP TIME: **15 min.**
TOTAL TIME: **6 hours**

Ingredients

- 2 cups dried small, white beans (navy beans), rinsed, soaked overnight and drained
- 4 cups water
- 2 bay leaves
- 3/4 teaspoon salt, divided
- 1 yellow onion, chopped
- 1/2 cup light molasses
- 1 1/2 tablespoons dry mustard
- 3 strips thick-cut bacon, cut into 1/2-inch pieces

Instructions

1. In a Dutch oven or a large ovenproof pot with a tight-fitting lid, combine beans, water, bay leaves and 1/2 teaspoon of the salt over high heat. Bring to a boil. Reduce heat to low, partially cover and simmer for 65 to 75 minutes until beans have softened but are firm. Remove from heat and discard bay leaves. Don't drain beans.
2. Preheat oven to 350°F (175°C).
3. Stir the onion, molasses, mustard, bacon and the remaining 1/4 teaspoon salt into the beans. Cover and bake for 4 1/2 to 5 hours until beans are tender and coated with a light syrup. Check periodically to make sure the beans don't dry out, stirring and adding hot water when needed.

Grilled Mango Chutney

SERVINGS: **6**
PREP TIME: **10 min.**
TOTAL TIME: **20 min.**

Ingredients

- 1 mango, peeled and pitted
- 1/4 cup sugar
- 1/4 cup chopped red onion
- 2 tablespoons cider vinegar
- 2 tablespoons finely chopped green bell pepper
- 1 tablespoon grated fresh ginger

- 1/2 teaspoon ground ginger
- 1/8 teaspoon ground cloves
- 1/4 teaspoon chopped fresh rosemary

Instructions

1. Preheat a gas grill or broiler. Position the cooking rack 4 to 6 inches from heat source.
2. Arrange mango on the grill rack or broiler pan. Broil on medium heat, about 2 to 3 minutes on each side, turning often, until softened and slightly browned.
3. Remove mango from the grill and let cool for a few minutes.
4. Chop small chunks and serve.

Sherried Mushroom Sauce

SERVINGS: **12**
PREP TIME: **5 min.**
TOTAL TIME: **20 min.**

Ingredients

- 2 cups fat-free milk
- 2 teaspoons canola oil
- 1 small onion, diced
- 1 1/2 cups sliced fresh mushrooms
- 2 tablespoons all-purpose (plain) flour
- 1 tablespoon chopped chives
- Ground black pepper, to taste
- 1 teaspoon sherry (optional)

Instructions

1. Over low heat, warm milk in a small saucepan.
2. Heat canola oil in a non-stick skillet over medium heat. Add onions and sauté for 3 minutes. Add sliced mushrooms and sauté another 3 minutes. Stir in flour and cook another 2 to 3 minutes. Whisk in warmed milk and stirring frequently until thickened, about 3 minutes. Add chives, pepper and sherry, if desired.
3. Keep mushroom sauce warmed over low heat until served.

Bulgur Stuffing with Dried Cranberries and Hazelnuts

SERVINGS: **10**
PREP TIME: **15 min.**
TOTAL TIME: **45 min.**

Ingredients
- 1 tablespoons olive oil
- 3 cups chopped onions (2 large)
- 1 cup chopped celery (2-3 stalks)
- 1 clove garlic, minced
- 1/2 teaspoon ground cinnamon
- 1/4 teaspoon ground allspice
- 2 cups bulgur, rinsed
- 3 cups reduced-sodium chicken broth
- 1 bay leaf
- 1/4 teaspoon salt

- 2/3 cup dried cranberries
- 1/4 cup orange juice
- 2/3 cup chopped hazelnuts (about 2 ounces) roasted
- 1/2 cup chopped fresh flat leaf parsley
- 1/4 teaspoon fresh ground black pepper

Instructions

1. Heat oil over medium heat. Add onions and celery, cook for 5-8 minutes stirring often until softened.
2. Add garlic, cinnamon and allspice, cook for one minute while stirring.
3. Add bulgur and stir for a few seconds, add broth, bay leaf and salt, bring to a simmer.
4. Reduce heat to low, cover and simmer 15-20 minutes until bulgur is tender and liquid is absorbed.
5. Meanwhile, combine dried cranberries and orange juice in a small microwave safe container. Cover with plastic wrap and microwave on high for 2 minutes. Let cranberries rest while covered, for another minute or two.
6. When bulgur has cooked, discard bay leaf, add cranberries with orange juice, toasted hazelnuts, parsley and pepper. Fluff with a fork and serve.

Southwest Potato Skins

SERVINGS: **6**
PREP TIME: **10 min.**
TOTAL TIME: **30 min.**

Ingredients

- 6 large baking potatoes
- 1 teaspoon olive oil
- 1 teaspoon chili powder
- 1/8 teaspoon Tabasco sauce
- 6 slices turkey bacon, cooked until crisp, chopped
- 1 medium tomato, diced
- 2 tablespoons sliced green onions
- 1/2 cup shredded cheddar cheese

Instructions

1. Preheat the oven to 450°F (230°F). Lightly coat a baking sheet with cooking spray.
2. Scrub potatoes and prick each several times with a fork. Microwave uncovered on high about 10 minutes or until tender. Remove potatoes from microwave and place on a wire rack to cool. When cool, cut each in half lengthwise. Scoop out the flesh, leaving about 1/4 inch of the flesh attached to the skin. (Save potato flesh for something else.)
3. Whisk together olive oil, chili powder and hot sauce in a small bowl. Brush olive oil mix on the insides of the potato skins. Cut each half of the potato skin in half crosswise again. Place potatoes on baking sheet.
4. Mix the turkey bacon, tomato and onions in a small bowl. Fill each potato skin with this mix and sprinkle with cheese.

5. Bake about 10 minutes or until cheese is melted and the potato skins are heated through.
6. Serve immediately.

Shrimp ceviche
SERVINGS: 8
PREP/TOTAL TIME: 10 min. + refrigeration

Ingredients
- 1/2 pound raw shrimp, cut in 1/4-inch pieces
- 2 lemons, zest and juice
- 2 limes, zest and juice
- 2 tablespoons olive oil
- 2 teaspoons cumin
- 1/2 cup diced red onion
- 1 cup diced tomato
- 2 tablespoons minced garlic
- 1 cup black beans, cooked
- 1/4 cup serrano chili pepper, diced and seeds removed
- 1 cup diced cucumber, peeled and seeded
- 1/4 cup chopped cilantro

Instructions
1. Place shrimp in a shallow pan and cover with juice from the lemon and lime. Reserving the zest. Refrigerate for at least 3 hours or until shrimp is firm and white.

2. In a separate bowl, mix remaining ingredients and set aside while shrimp is cooking in the fridge. When ready to serve, mix shrimp and citrus juice with remaining ingredients.
3. Serve with tortilla chips.

PART 2

INTRODUCTION

This book contains proven steps and strategies on how to prepare a week's worth of meals without having the need to add sodium.

Technically speaking, there are several eating plans that were released over the years but this particular plan is what you really need to lower your risks of having a heart condition or if you were already diagnosed with one, ways on how you can live your life to the fullest in terms of food consumption. DASH diet means Dietary Approaches to Stop Hypertension.

Doctors observed that more and more people are eating the wrong kind of food. Fast food joints are everywhere and most are open 24 hours a day and fast-paced corporate life seem easier with food-on-the-go.

How can one consume that much sodium? You have to thank the chips, alcohol and energy drinks for that. 1 out of 4 adult Americans have high blood pressure because they blindly eat "feel-good" salty food and would rather sit than walk on a daily basis. This book has many suggested recipes based on a 14-day DASH diet menu that will help control hypertension, not leave you hungry and will keep your sodium levels at bay. But keep in mind that going on a strict diet plan without physical activity will not do the trick.

The first way to re-arrange your diet is to reduce your daily sodium intake to less than 2,300 mg. Starting on a diet meal plan that gained praises from doctors will help you start and reach your goal of feeling and looking your best. Did you know that the DASH diet was created to prevent elevated blood pressure from staying more elevated? The best way to prevent it is to eat low-sodium food. It may be difficult to live on a no-sodium diet since food would taste bland. If you should know, the common sodium intake nowadays is 3,500 to 5,000 mg. The right way to a man's heart is definitely through his stomach and this book will show you the way.

Thanks again for downloading this book, I hope you enjoy it!

CHAPTER 1. WHAT TO EAT IN A DASH DIET

The DASH diet is low in saturated fat, total fat and cholesterol. Following are the guidelines as well as suggested servings for each of the food groups within a daily 2,000 calorie DASH diet.

On Grains

Use whole grains instead of refined ones.
Use brown rice instead of white rice.
Use whole wheat pasta instead of regular pasta.
Use whole grain bread instead of regular bread.
Recommended serving is 6 to 8 a day.

On Vegetables

Frozen vegetables contain salt to prolong shelf-life; choose low-in sodium or without added salt products with a shorter shelf-life.
Reduce the amount of meat and load up on the vegetables.
Add spices instead of creams because most spices come with Vitamin D.
Recommended serving is 4 to 5 a day.

On Fruits

Canned fruits contain extra sugar; choose no added sugar or sugar-free instead.

Some pits add texture to meals and contain high levels of fiber.

Use fruits as a snack or part of a main course.

Some peels are edible, nutritious and comes packed with Vitamin C.

Recommended serving is 4 to 5 a day.

Natural Fat Source

Dairy products are rich in saturated fat; choose fat-free or low-fat products.

A cup of yogurt instead of plain milk can do wonders if you are lactose-intolerant.

Cheese is high in sodium; look for sodium-free hard cheese instead.

Recommended serving is 2 to 3 a day.

Lean Proteins

The best source of protein and B vitamins is meat but consumption should be in moderation.

Meat contains cholesterol but that doesn't mean that you have to completely avoid it; keep a small serving instead of making it the main meal of the day.

Bake, roast, or broil meat instead of fry, but if you must fry, use olive oil.

Fish comes with different fatty acids; choose tuna, herring and salmon which are high in omega-3 content that helps the body keep cholesterol levels low.

Recommended serving is 2 to 6 a day.

Where the Beans are

Seeds and nuts are some of the best sources of magnesium, protein and potassium (apart from meat).

Add to stir-fry meals, cereals and salads.

High calorie content restricts them to a weekly consumption.

Good substitute for protein are soybeans for they contain amino acids.

Recommended serving is 4 to 5 a day.

The Good, the Fat and the Oily

Fat absorbs essential vitamins and strengthens the immune system.

Too much fat leads to heart ailments; limit intake to 27 percent or less from daily calorie fat consumption.

Go against saturated fat and support monounsaturated fat.

Limit consumption of butter, cream, eggs, whole milk and meat.

Avoid processed food that contains oil and sodium.

Think soft margarines, mayonnaise and salad dressings.

Recommended serving is 2 to 3 a day.

Candies and Sweets

When craving for sweets, look for hard candy, low-fat cookies, sorbet, jelly beans.

Do not buy all products with the word "diet" attached to the labels; they contain artificial sweeteners.

Go for regular soda instead of diet soda but drink in moderation.

Recommended serving is 2 to 4 a day.

CHAPTER 2. DAY 1 MEAL PLAN WITH RECIPES

Breakfast - Low-Fat Blueberry Pancakes

Lunch - Shrimp with Mixed Greens Vinaigrette Salad

Dinner - Salmon with Orange and Mint Vinaigrette

Snacks (mid-day or before dinner) - Apple- Cinnamon Muffins with Ricotta Cheese

Breakfast: Low-Fat Blueberry Pancakes
Ingredients
1 and 1/3 cups buttermilk (low-fat)
1 cup all-purpose flour
2 teaspoons baking powder
1 tablespoon sugar
1 tablespoon vegetable oil
1/4 teaspoon baking soda
1/4 cup egg substitute
Cooking spray
Maple syrup (for topping)

1/2 cup frozen blueberries

Directions
- In a large bowl, combine the baking powder, all-purpose flour, baking soda and sugar.
- Add in the egg substitute, oil and buttermilk to the dry ingredients, stir in blueberries.
- Coat a skillet with cooking spray and pour ¼ cup of the batter.
- Transfer into a plate and drizzle maple syrup; serve with blueberries on the side.

Lunch: Shrimp with Mixed Greens Vinaigrette Salad

Ingredients
2 and 1/2 cups frozen red raspberries
12 endive leaves
1 package frozen baby corn
12 ounces fresh asparagus spears
1/4 cup wine vinegar
1/4 cup walnut oil
12 spinach leaves
12 ounces frozen shrimp
12 lettuce leaves
1 tablespoon fresh parsley
2 teaspoons honey

Directions
- In a skillet, cook shrimp, corn and asparagus in boiling water for 8 minutes; drain water and set aside.
- In a large bowl, toss the leafy vegetables and berries; pour the vinegar, walnut oil and honey dressing.
- Transfer the boiled vegetables to a plate and garnish with parsley.

DINNER: Salmon with Orange and Mint Vinaigrette

Ingredients
6 cups mixed greens
1 and 1/2 pounds fresh salmon fillet
1 tablespoon fresh basil
2 tablespoons onion
1/2 cup dry white wine
1 tablespoon orange peel
1/4 cup balsamic vinegar
1/3 cup fresh orange juice
1 tablespoon fresh mint
1/2 cup water
1 tablespoon fresh parsley

Directions
- In a jar with a lid, combine the orange juice, orange peel, vinegar, parsley, mint, basil, and onions; cover the lid, shake well and refrigerate.
- In a large skillet, bring water and white wine to a boil and add the sliced fish.
- Meanwhile, place the salad greens on a plate and place the fillet on top.
- Serve with the vinaigrette.

Snack: Apple- Cinnamon Fluffs with Ricotta Cheese

Ingredients

1 tablespoon vanilla extract

1 teaspoon baking soda

1 cup low-fat buttermilk

3 tablespoons sugar

1 tablespoon baking powder

3 tablespoons vegetable oil

Cooking spray

1 large egg

2 teaspoons ground cinnamon

2 large egg whites

1 and 1/2 cups apple

1 cup sugar

1/3 cup 2% low-fat milk

2 teaspoons ground cinnamon

1/3 cup light ricotta cheese

2 and 1/3 cups all-purpose flour

Directions

- Preheat your oven to 400 degrees F.
- In a large bowl, combine the sugar, baking powder, all-purpose flour, shredded apple, baking soda and cinnamon.
- Add buttermilk, vanilla, cheese, egg whites vegetable oil, and egg.

- When the wet ingredients are mixed, combine it with the dry ingredients and stir until the mixture moistens.
- Prepare a muffin pan, grease with cooking spray and pour the batter.
- Coat the batter with cinnamon and sugar on top then bake in the oven for about 18 minutes.
- Once the muffin fluffs are done, remove them from the pan and serve.

CHAPTER 3. DAY 2 MEAL PLAN WITH RECIPES

Breakfast - Quick Power-up Banana Smoothie

Lunch - Grilled Beef with Salad Greens in Avocado-Lime Vinaigrette

Dinner - Almond-Parmesan Crusted Fish with Tartar Sauce

Snacks (mid-day or before dinner) - Wheat-Bran Cinnamon Cereal Muffins

Breakfast: Quick Power-up Banana Smoothie

Ingredients
1/2 cup 1% low-fat milk
1/2 cup crushed ice
1 tablespoon honey
1 large ripe banana
1 carton vanilla fat-free yogurt

Directions
- In a blender, add banana, low-fat milk, crushed ice and honey; blend until smooth.

- Pour honey on top, stir the smoothie with a spoon; transfer into a tall glass and enjoy!

Lunch: Grilled Beef with Salad Greens in Avocado-Lime Vinaigrette

Ingredients
6 cups torn mixed salad greens
1 small avocado
1/2 cup Italian salad dressing (reduced-calorie)
2 tablespoons fresh cilantro
1/4 teaspoon ground black pepper
1/2 teaspoon lime peel (finely shredded)
1/4 cup onion (chopped)
2 small yellow tomatoes
1/4 cup lime juice
12 ounces beef flank steak

Directions
- Preheat your oven to 160 degrees F.
- In a zip-lock bag, insert the steak and place it on a shallow dish; set aside.
- In a screw-lid jar, combine the dressing by mixing the lime peel, salad dressing and cilantro; cover and shake.
- In a small bowl, pour half of the dressing mixture and refrigerate for 5 minutes.
- In the jar, add the onions; cover and shake then add with the steal; marinate overnight.
- The following day, remove the bag from the refrigerator and discard the marinade.

- Transfer the steak on a broiler pan; sprinkle with pepper.
- Broil the steak in the oven for 18 minutes or depending on your preferred doneness.
- Once done, remove the steak from the oven and transfer on a chopping board to slice it across the grain.
- On a plate, arrange the salad green, avocado slices and tomatoes; top with the steak.
- Drizzle the remaining salad dressing and serve.

Dinner: Almond-Parmesan Crusted Fish with Tartar Sauce

Ingredients
1 pound fresh fish fillets
2 tablespoons butter (unsalted)
2 tablespoons milk
1 beaten egg
2 tablespoons ground almonds
1/4 cup finely round crackers
2 tablespoons grated Parmesan cheese
1/8 teaspoon pepper
1/2 teaspoon dried basil
Tartar Sauce

Directions
- Preheat your oven to 500 degrees F.
- In a shallow dish, combine the milk and egg.
- In another dish, combine the parmesan cheese, ground crackers, basil, ground nuts, pepper and basil.
- Dip the fish in in the egg mixture and roll in the crumb mixture.
- In a baking pan, melt butter and add the breaded fish.
- Transfer the pan in the oven and bake for 15 minutes until the fish turns flaky.

- Meanwhile, to make the tartar sauce, stir salad dressing, chopped dill pickle, parsley, diced pimiento, lemon juice and sliced green onions in a small bowl.
- Serve the fish and transfer the sauce into a dipping dish and enjoy!

Snack: Wheat-Bran Cinnamon Cereal Muffins

Ingredients
1 teaspoon baking soda
1 and 3/4 cups all-purpose flour
Cooking spray
2 tablespoons butter
1 can crushed pineapple
3/4 cup milk (fat-free)
1 cup shredded carrot
1 teaspoon ground cinnamon
1 cup wheat bran flakes cereal
2 tablespoons water
1/4 cup sugar
1 teaspoon baking powder
1 large egg

Directions
- Preheat your oven to 350 degrees F.
- Prepare the muffin tin cups by greasing it with cooking spray.
- In a large bowl, mix together the baking powder, all-purpose flour, cinnamon, baking soda and sugar.
- In a large bowl, add the cereal mixture, flour mixture and carrots then spoon them in muffin cups.
- In a small bowl, combine the beaten egg, milk, cereals, crushed pineapples with juice and the butter; set it aside for five minutes.

- In a small saucepan, bring the carrots and water to a boil then remove when carrots soften.
- Drain the saucepan from water and set aside the carrots in a small plate.
- Pop the muffin cups in the oven for 22 minutes until it turns golden brown.
- Remove the muffins, garnish with carrot shreds and cinnamon powder; serve the Wheat-Bran Cinnamon Cereal Muffins.

CHAPTER 4. DAY 3 MEAL PLAN WITH RECIPES

Breakfast

Buttermilk Baked Whole-grain Biscuits
1 cup of Almonds

Lunch
Grilled Chicken over Vinaigrette Greens Salad Sliced Bell Peppers
1 cup Sugar-free gelatin (store-bought)

Dinner - Almond-Parmesan Crusted Fish with Tartar Sauce

Snacks (mid-day or before dinner) - Bacon and Broccoli Egg Muffin

Breakfast: Buttermilk Baked Whole-grain Biscuits

Ingredients
¾ cup all-purpose flour
1/2 teaspoon bicarbonate soda
2 teaspoons baking powder

3 tablespoons wheat germ
1 cup low-fat buttermilk
1 cup whole-wheat flour
3 tablespoons butter

Directions
- Preheat your oven to 400 degrees F and one ungreased baking sheet.
- In a bowl, combine the all-purpose flour, whole-wheat flour, butter and bicarbonate soda.
- Add buttermilk to the dry mixture to create the dough; cover the bowl with plastic and refrigerate for about 30 minutes.
- Dust your clean tabletop with all-purpose flour and knead the chilled dough.
- With a rolling pin, roll out the dough and cut into half an inch thick rectangles.
- Arrange the unbaked biscuits on your ungreased cookie sheet and bake in the oven for 10 minutes.
- Once the biscuits are done, transfer into a plate and serve hot.

Lunch: Grilled Chicken over Vinaigrette Greens Salad

Ingredients
1 package torn mixed greens
3 cloves garlic
3/4 cup balsamic vinaigrette salad dressing (bottled)
4 pieces of chicken breast
1/4 teaspoon red pepper (crushed)

Directions
- In a zip-lock bag, add the chicken breast and vinaigrette, garlic and crushed red peppers; shake well and refrigerate the marinade for 4 hours.
- Drain the chicken after four hours; reserve the marinade.
- Transfer the chicken to an uncovered grill and grill for about 15 minutes; discard the marinade.
- On a large serving plate, arrange the salad greens and top with the grilled chicken strips.
- Pour the remaining ¼ cup of vinaigrette and serve.

Dinner: Almond-Parmesan Crusted Fish with Tartar Sauce

Ingredients
1 pound fresh fish fillets
2 tablespoons butter (unsalted)
2 tablespoons milk
1 beaten egg
2 tablespoons ground almonds
1/4 cup finely round crackers
2 tablespoons grated Parmesan cheese
1/8 teaspoon pepper
1/2 teaspoon dried basil
Tartar Sauce

Directions
- Preheat your oven to 500 degrees F.
- In a shallow dish, combine the milk and egg.
- In another dish, combine the parmesan cheese, ground crackers, basil, ground nuts, pepper and basil.
- Dip the fish in in the egg mixture and roll in the crumb mixture.
- In a baking pan, melt butter and add the breaded fish.
- Transfer the pan in the oven and bake for 15 minutes until the fish turns flaky.

- Meanwhile, to make the tartar sauce, stir salad dressing, chopped dill pickle, parsley, diced pimiento, lemon juice and sliced green onions in a small bowl.
- Serve the fish and transfer the sauce into a dipping dish and enjoy!

Snack: Bacon and Broccoli Egg Muffin

Ingredients
1 small bunch of spinach
¼ cup sliced and diced mushrooms
6 strips of cooked bacon
1/2 cup broccoli
12 eggs
Cooking spray (vegetable oil)
1 small bell pepper

Directions
- Heat the oven at 350 degrees F.
- Line muffin tins with cooking spray.
- In a skillet, add the bacon strips and cook it to a crisp.
- Once the bacon is done, chop into little pieces.
- Break 12 eggs and mix with the broccoli, pepper, bacon, spinach and mushrooms.
- In a colander, rinse and drain the broccoli before cutting it into little pieces.
- Pour the egg mix into the muffin tin and bake in the oven for about 25 minutes.
- When cooked, garnish the muffins with a few bacon slices and serve.

CHAPTER 5. DAY 4 MEAL PLAN WITH

RECIPES

Breakfast - White Tuna Pita Pockets with Romaine Lettuce

Lunch - Pesto Tortellini with Broccoli

Dinner - Authentic Asian 5-Spice Roasted Duck Breast

Snacks (mid-day or before dinner) - Carrot- Pineapple Muffins with Bran Flakes

BREAKFAST: White Tuna Pita Pockets with Romaine Lettuce

-
Ingredients
1/2 cup green bell peppers (finely chopped)
3/4 cup diced tomatoes
1 and 1/2 cups romaine lettuce
1/2 cup broccoli (finely chopped)
1/2 cup shredded carrots
2 cans white tuna in water (low-salt)
1/4 cup onion (finely chopped)
3 pita pockets (whole-wheat)

1/2 cup ranch dressing (low-fat)

Directions
- In a large bowl, add the tomatoes, carrots, lettuce, broccoli, peppers, and onions; toss everything.
- In a small bowl, combine the ranch dressing, tuna mixture and lettuce.
- Scoop the tuna salad and fill each pita pocket; serve immediately.

Lunch: Pesto Tortellini with Broccoli

Ingredients
1 cup heavy cream
¼ cup pesto (bottled)
¼ cup Parmesan cheese
12 ounces tortellini pasta
1 cups broccoli (steamed)

Directions
- In a large pot, bring water to a boil then add the broccoli and tortellini pasta.
- Cook the vegetables for about 15 minutes until the broccoli is tender and pasta is al dente.
- In a saucepan, simmer the pesto sauce and a cup of heavy cream; stir until thickened.
- Remove from the heat and dust parmesan cheese on top before tossing with pasta and broccoli.
- Serve the pesto tortellini with garlic bread on the side and enjoy!

Dinner: Authentic Asian 5-Spice Roasted Duck Breast

Ingredients
2 teaspoons honey
2 pounds boneless duck breast
2 oranges (Zest & juice)
1 teaspoon five-spice powder
1/4 teaspoon cornstarch
1 tablespoon soy sauce (reduced-sodium)

Directions
- Preheat your oven to 375 degrees F.
- Place the duck on a cutting board with its skin-side facing down.
- Trim off excess skin and make diagonal cuts; sprinkle 5-Spice powder.
- In a skillet, place the duck and cook until golden brown; transfer to oven.
- Roast the duck for 15 minutes; once done, transfer to a cutting board to rest for 5 minutes.
- In the same skillet, pour the duck fat from the pan and simmer with honey and orange juice.
- Add in the soy sauce and orange zest and cook until sauce is reduced.
- Add in the cornstarch and stir until mixture is thick.
- Transfer the duck to a plate, thinly sliced it and serve with the orange sauce.

Ingredients for the 5-Spice Seasoning
1 and 1⁄2teaspoons fennel seeds
6 pieces of star anise
3⁄4 teaspoon ground cloves
3 tablespoons cinnamon
1 and 1⁄2 teaspoons whole black peppercorns

Directions for the 5-Spice Seasoning
- Combine all the ingredients in blender until they are finely ground.

Snack: Carrot- Pineapple Muffins with Bran Flakes

Ingredients
3/4 cup milk (fat-free)
1 and 3/4 cups all-purpose flour
1 teaspoon baking powder
1/4 cup sugar
1 large egg
1 cup wheat bran flakes cereal
1 teaspoon ground cinnamon
1 teaspoon baking soda
1 can crushed pineapple in juice
2 tablespoons of butter (unsalted)
2 tablespoons water
Cooking spray
1 cup shredded carrot

Directions
- Preheat your oven to 350 degrees F; grease muffin cups with cooking spray.
- In a small saucepan, boil the chopped carrots until tender; set aside.
- Meanwhile, combine the sugar, baking powder, ground cinnamon, baking soda and all-purpose flour in a large bowl.
- Add the fat-free milk, egg, cereals and the crushed pineapple juice; stir well.

- Add the tender carrots and mix to combine all ingredients.
- Spoon the carrot batter in to the muffin pan and place in the oven to bake for 20 minutes.
- Once the muffins are done, allow it to set on the pan for 5 minutes; transfer on a wire rack to cool.
- Serve your homemade muffins as a snack before lunch time or dinner time.

Chapter 6. Day 5 Meal Plan with Recipes

Breakfast - Ham and Egg Sandwich on Toasted Muffins

Lunch
Cajun-Breaded Fish & Chips
1 cup Sugar-free gelatin (store-bought)

Dinner - Chili Mahi-Mahi Fillet with Balsamic Spinach Salad

Snacks (mid-day or before dinner) - Goat Cheese-Bell Pepper Frittata

Breakfast: Ham and Egg Sandwich on Toasted Muffins

-
Ingredients
Vegetable cooking spray (store-bought)
1 whole-wheat muffin (store-bought)
1 slice Swiss cheese
1 tablespoon apricot preserves
2 slices deli ham
Freshly ground pepper (for sprinkling)

1 large egg

Directions
- Coat a skillet with cooking spray to lightly brown 2 slices of ham.
- Top the cooked ham and melted cheese; set aside.
- In the same skillet, fry one egg and cook it sunny-side up.
- Cut the muffins in the middle and toast until lightly brown.
- Spread apricot preserves on the toasted muffins; layer the ham and eggs; sprinkle freshly ground pepper and serve.

Lunch: Cajun-Breaded Fish & Chips

Ingredients
1 pound cod
1/4 cup all-purpose flour
2 large egg whites
1 and 1/2 pound russet potatoes
1 and 1/2 teaspoon Cajun seasoning
4 teaspoons olive oil
2 cups cornflakes
Cooking spray

Directions
- Preheat your oven to 425 degrees F and coat a baking sheet with cooking spray; set aside.
- In a large bowl, toss the potatoes with oil and Cajun seasoning.
- In a food processor, coarsely grind the cornflakes; transfer to a shallow dish together with the flour.
- In another shallow dish, mix egg whites and Cajun seasoning for dredging.
- Dip the cod fish in the cornflakes and dredge in egg white mixture.
- Place potatoes and fish on the baking sheet and bake in the oven for 35 minutes.
- Once done, serve the fish and potatoes chips on a plate and enjoy!

Dinner: Chili Mahi-Mahi Fillet with Balsamic Spinach Salad

Ingredients
1 pound mahi-mahi
1 onion
1/4 teaspoon pepper
1 teaspoon olive oil
4 cups baby spinach (chopped)
2 tablespoons cooking oil
1 small yellow sweet pepper
4 tablespoons red jalapeno jelly
1 tablespoon balsamic vinegar

Directions
- In a large bowl, place chopped baby spinach; set aside.
- In a skillet, cook the jalapeno jelly, sweet pepper and spinach with oil; set aside.
- Meanwhile, cut the mahi-mahi fillets into serving-sized pieces; sprinkle with pepper.
- Cook the mahi-mahi fillet in olive oil for about 5 minutes until flaky; transfer to a platter.
- In the same skillet, cook the jalapeno jelly and spread over the mahi-mahi.

- Serve the fish with balsamic spinach salad and enjoy!

Snack: Goat Cheese-Bell Pepper Frittata

Ingredients
  1 cup red bell pepper (sliced)
1/4 teaspoon ground pepper
1 bunch scallions (sliced)
2 tablespoons olive oil (extra-virgin)
8 eggs 1/2 cup goat cheese (crumbled)
2 tablespoons oregano

Directions
- Preheat your boiler and prepare a large skillet.
- In a medium-sized bowl, add pepper, whisked eggs and oregano.
- In the skillet, add the scallions and bell pepper and cook for 30 seconds until they wilt.
- Combine the egg mixture with the wilted vegetables for 3 minutes to create a frittata.
- Sprinkle cheese over the cooked frittata and broil it in the skillet for 3 minutes until they eggs fluff up.
- Allow the Goat Cheese, Bell Pepper and Oregano Frittata to rest for 3 minutes before you serve it on a plate.

CHAPTER **7.** DAY **6** MEAL PLAN WITH RECIPES

Breakfast
Hot Tomato Pan-Fried Eggs
1 cup of grapes

Lunch
Hot Tomato Pan-Fried Eggs
1 cup Sugar-free gelatin (store-bought)

Dinner - Garlic-Broccoli Rigatoni Pasta

Snacks (mid-day or before dinner) - Homemade French Toasts in Sugar, Cinnamon

Breakfast: Hot Tomato Pan-Fried Eggs

Ingredients
1 garlic clove
2 large zucchinis
200g cherry tomatoes
1 tbsp. olive oil
¼ tsp. cayenne pepper

Basil leaves (for garnish)
2 eggs

Directions
- In a frying pan, cook the sliced zucchinis in olive oil for about 5 minutes.
- Add garlic, tomatoes in the pan and sauté for a few minutes; set aside.
- Crack the eggs directly on the pan and cook for 3 minutes.
- Transfer the Hot Tomato Pan-Fried Eggs and garnish with basil leaves.

Lunch: Hot Tomato Pan-Fried Eggs

Ingredients
1 garlic clove
2 large zucchinis
200g cherry tomatoes
1 tbsp. olive oil
¼ tsp. cayenne pepper
Basil leaves (for garnish)
2 eggs

Directions
- In a frying pan, cook the sliced zucchinis in olive oil for about 5 minutes.
- Add garlic, tomatoes in the pan and sauté for a few minutes; set aside.
- Crack the eggs directly on the pan and cook for 3 minutes.
- Transfer the Hot Tomato Pan-Fried Eggs and garnish with basil leaves.

Dinner: Garlic-Broccoli Rigatoni Pasta

Ingredients
1 cup broccoli florets
2 teaspoons garlic (minced)
2 tablespoons Parmesan cheese

2 teaspoons olive oil
1/3 pound rigatoni noodles
Black pepper (freshly ground)

Directions
- In a large pot, bring water to a boil and add the pasta; cook until al dente.
- Meanwhile, in another pot, steam the broccoli florets for about 10 minutes.
- After 12 minutes, drain pasta in a colander; set aside.
- Combine and toss broccoli and pasta with grated parmesan cheese, garlic and olive oil.
- Sprinkle freshly ground black pepper; immediately serve on a plate and enjoy!

-

Snack: Homemade French Toasts in Sugar, Cinnamon

Ingredients
2 eggs and 1 yolk
1 and 3/4 cups milk
1/2 cup granulated sugar
1 tsp vanilla extract
4 tablespoons of butter
12 slices of whole grain bread

Directions
- In a medium-sized bowl, mix the yolk, eggs, vanilla and sugar.
- In a large skillet, heat butter and sprinkle sugar to caramelize.
- Immerse a slice of whole grain bread in the milk mixture and place in the pan.
- Keep adding sugar to both sides and cook until golden.
- Serve the French toast on a plate and sprinkle cinnamon and nutmeg.

CHAPTER 8. DAY 7 MEAL PLAN WITH RECIPES

Breakfast - Baked Breakfast Sausages in Rosemary and Olive Oil

Lunch
Baked Cheesy Potatoes with Mushrooms
1 cup Sugar-free gelatin (store-bought)

Dinner - Chicken with Pepper-Garlic, Tarragon and Leeks

Snacks (mid-day or before dinner) - Pineapple-Flavored Carrot Bran Muffins

Breakfast: Baked Breakfast Sausages in Rosemary and Olive Oil

Ingredients
1 package breakfast sausages
1 teaspoon fresh rosemary
1 medium onion
2 teaspoons whole grain mustard
1 tablespoon olive oil
Fresh rosemary sprigs (for garnishing)

Freshly ground black pepper

Directions

- Preheat your oven to 500 degrees F and prepare an ungreased baking sheet.
- In a small skillet, sauté chopped rosemary leaves, onions in olive oil; set aside in a bowl.
- In the same skillet, add ground pepper, mustard and sausages with casings.
- Mix the sausage mixture and form into patties; transfer to a baking sheet.
- Transfer the baking sheet in the oven and bake for 6 minutes.
- Remove to blot excess oil on paper towels and serve on a platter.
- Garnish the breakfast sausages with rosemary sprigs and serve.

Lunch: Baked Cheesy Potatoes with Mushrooms

Ingredients
1/2 cup dried mushrooms
1 small onion
1 tablespoon olive oil
2 tablespoons all-purpose flour
1/8 teaspoon pepper
1 1/4 cups skim milk
½ cup Parmesan cheese
3 baking potatoes

Directions
- In a small bowl, pour warm water and add the mushrooms; keep it covered and soak for 30 minutes.
- Once the mushrooms are tender, drain the water from the bowl and coarsely chop the mushrooms.
- In a skillet, sauté the onions and mushrooms until tender; stir in the flour, milk and pepper.
- Cook the mushrooms mixture until it thickens; stir in half of the grated parmesan cheese.
- Meanwhile, grease a casserole with oil and add half of the sliced potatoes and half of the sauce.
- Repeat the process of layering until the casserole is full and sprinkle the remainder of the cheese on top.

- Place the casserole in the oven and bake for 35 minutes with a cover.
- Once the potato casserole is tender and golden brown, allow to cool at room temperature before serving.

-

Dinner: Chicken with Pepper-Garlic, Tarragon and Leeks

Ingredients
8 ounces chicken breast
2 leeks
1 small onion
3 garlic cloves
2 cups chicken broth (low-sodium)
1 teaspoon olive oil (extra-virgin)
1 cup frozen peas
2/3 cup brown rice
2 large tomatoes
1 teaspoon tarragon
1 red pepper
1 lemon wedges (quartered)
1/4 cup fresh parsley (chopped)

Directions
- In a large frying pan, sauté garlic, leeks, chicken strips and onions in olive oil.
- Add the tarragon, chicken broth, brown rice, red pepper slices and tomatoes for another 15 minutes.
- Stir in the peas and continue to simmer to cook the rice; remove pan from heat after about 60 minutes.
- Serve the chicken and vegetables on a plate; garnish with a lemon wedge parsley.

Snack) Pineapple-Flavored Carrot Bran Muffins

Ingredients
2 tablespoons butter
3/4 cup milk (fat-free)
1 and 3/4 cups all-purpose flour
1 teaspoon baking powder
1/4 cup sugar
1 teaspoon baking soda
1 can crushed pineapple in juice
1 large egg
1 teaspoon ground cinnamon
1 cup wheat bran flakes cereal
2 tablespoons water
1 cup shredded carrot
Cooking spray

Directions
- Preheat your oven to 350 degrees F and grease a muffin tin with cooking spray.
- In a large bowl, combine flour, sugar, baking powder and baking powder.
- Once you have fully combined the flour mixture, add the sugar, milk, cereal and cinnamon to the bowl, set aside for 5 minutes.
- Meanwhile, in a small saucepan, add water and carrot and bring to a boil.
- Once the carrots are tender, drain the water and set aside.

- Add the carrots to the flour mixture and stir until moist.
- Spoon in batter to the muffin tin and bake in the oven for about 22 minutes or until it turn golden brown.
- Once cooked, remove the muffins from the pan and immediately serve.

CHAPTER **9**. DASH DIET ALL-DAY RECIPES

Here are additional Dash Diet recipes that you can prepare all day. The meal plan is good for 7 days and beyond that, you can continue on with the Dash Diet. These simple meals can also serve 4-6 people.

Spiced Walnuts and Apples Oatmeal

Ingredients
1 teaspoon ground cloves
1 cup chopped dried dates
2 tablespoons ground cinnamon
1 cup chopped walnuts
1 cup brown sugar
1 teaspoon ground turmeric
1 cup chopped dried apples
3 cups grain cereal flakes
1 tablespoon ground ginger
3 cups rolled oats

Direction
- In a large bowl, combine the dates, oats, cereal, walnuts, apples, brown sugar, cloves, turmeric and ginger.

- In a microwave, boil one cup of water and pour it over the large bowl.
- Stir the oatmeal mix and make sure every dry ingredient is softened and let it stand for 10 minutes before serving.

Baked Beef Sausage Ciabatta

Ingredients
8 ounces Ciabatta bread
1 cup sharp cheddar cheese (reduced fat)
1/2 cup green onions
1 lb. beef breakfast sausage
1 and 1/4 cups fat-free milk
1 carton egg substitute
Cooking spray
2 tablespoons fresh parsley
2 large eggs

Directions
- Preheat your oven to 400 degrees F.
- On a baking sheet, line the Ciabatta bread cubes in one layer and bake in the oven for 8 minutes.
- As soon as the bread turns golden brown, remove from it from the oven and set aside to cool.
- Coat cooking spray and add the sausages cook in a small pan,
- In the same pan, add beaten eggs, cheese, egg substitute and milk.
- Meanwhile, combine the egg mixture with the bread mixture; set aside.
- In a baking dish, coat it with cooking spray and refrigerate for about 8 hours.
- After eight hours, preheat your oven once more for 350 degrees F and bake the casserole for 50 minutes.

- Once it is ready, remove the baking dish and serve.

-

Quick Spinach Omelet

Ingredients
1 recipe red pepper relish
Cooking spray
2 tablespoons chives
8 eggs
 2 cups spinach leaves
1/8 teaspoon cayenne pepper
1/2 cup cheddar cheese

Ingredients for the Red Pepper Relish
2 tablespoons green onion
2/3 cup red sweet pepper
1 tablespoon cider vinegar
1/4 teaspoon black pepper

Directions
- In a skillet, spray cooking oil and combine the chives, egg and cayenne pepper.
- When the eggs are cooked, add the cheddar cheese, spinach and pepper relish.
- As soon as the spinach leaves have wilted, transfer the omelet into a plate and top with the pepper relish and enjoy your Quick Spinach Omelet.

Directions for the Red Pepper Relish
- Prepare a small bowl and add the green onion, red sweet pepper, ground black pepper and cider vinegar.

- Toss all the ingredients in a small bowl and set aside to use for topping.

Crusted Mozzarella Chicken Nuggets

Ingredients
1 cup almond flour
2 eggs
1/2 cup coconut oil
2 chicken breasts
onion powder
pepper
1/2 cup mozzarella cheese
Garlic powder

Directions
- Season the chicken nuggets with onion powder, garlic powder and pepper.
- Dip chicken nuggets into scrambled egg batter.
- In a separate plate, roll the nuggets on the cheese and almond flour mix.
- In a saucepan, prepare the chicken nuggets with coconut oil for 3 minutes until it turns golden brown.
- Serve right away and garnish with parsley.

Ranch Chicken Fajita Wraps

Ingredients
1 small green sweet pepper
12 ounces chicken breast strips
1/3 cup cheddar cheese (reduced-fat)
1/4 teaspoon garlic powder
2 10-inch whole wheat tortillas
2 tablespoons ranch salad dressing (reduced-calorie)
Cooking spray
1/2 teaspoon chili powder
1/2 cup Fresh Salsa

Directions
- Preheat your oven to 350 degrees F.
- In a medium-sized skillet, spray cooking oil and add the chicken strips, garlic powder and chili powder.
- Cook the ingredients for about 6 minutes to remove the rawness of the chicken and to soften the sweet peppers.
- Once done, transfer the pepper and chicken to a plate and set aside.
- Line the tortillas in the oven for 10 minutes until it blisters and heats up.
- Remove when done and transfer to a plate.
- Get the chicken and red green peppers, sprinkle a handful of cheddar cheese and place it on the warm tortilla.
- Wrap the tortilla in a foil and place it back in the oven.

Ingredients for the Fresh Salsa Dip
1/4 cup green sweet pepper
1/4 cup red onion
2 tomatoes
1/2 teaspoon minced garlic
3 teaspoons cilantro
Black pepper
Hot pepper sauce (for added flavor)

Directions for the Fresh Salsa Dip
- In a medium bowl, add the minced red onions, tomatoes, garlic, cilantro and drop of hot sauce.
- Combine the ingredients together to make a salsa and chill for 30 minutes before serving.
- Serve the with Ranch Chicken Fajita Wraps and enjoy!

Stir-Fry Beef with Broccoli and Ginger

Ingredients
8 ounces beef top round steak
1/2 cup beef broth (reduced-sodium)
3 tablespoons soy sauce (reduced-sodium)
2-1/2 teaspoons cornstarch
1 teaspoon sugar
1/2 teaspoon fresh ginger
Cooking spray
12 ounces fresh or frozen asparagus
1-1/2 cups sliced fresh mushrooms
1 cup small broccoli florets
4 green onions
2 teaspoons olive oil
2 cups cooked brown rice

Directions
- Start this recipe by trimming off excess fat from the round steak.
- Prepare the sauce by getting a small bowl to mix the cornstarch, soy sauce, sugar, ginger and beef broth.
- Set the first few ingredients aside and cook the vegetables.
- Coat a large skillet with cooking oil and add the mushrooms, green onions, broccoli florets and asparagus.
- Cook for about 5 minutes to soften the vegetables then once done, serve on a plate.

- In the same skillet, add the meat and olive oil; stir-fry the sliced round steak for 3 minutes, add the sauce and cook until done.
- Get the plate you set aside and add all the vegetables in the skillet.
- Cook for 2 minutes to heat the sauce.
- Serve the Stir-Fry Beef with Broccoli and Ginger on top of cooked rice.

Spicy Meatballs with Cilantro and Parsley

Ingredients for the Meatballs
1 egg
1 pound ground beef
1 small finely chopped onion
1/4 teaspoon ground ginger
2 tablespoons fresh cilantro (minced)
1 tablespoon paprika
3 tablespoons fresh parsley (minced)
2 tablespoons ground cumin
1/4 teaspoon cayenne pepper
1/2 teaspoon cinnamon
1/2 teaspoon pepper
Ingredients for the Sauce
1 cup of beef broth (organic)
2 tablespoons olive oil
2 cups crushed organic tomatoes
2 medium chopped onions
1/2 teaspoon black pepper

1/2 cup parsley (freshly chopped)
4 minced garlic cloves
2 teaspoons ground cumin
1/2 cup parsley (freshly chopped)
Pinch of cayenne

Directions

- In a large bowl, mix all meatball ingredients and roll them into large balls.
- Drizzle coconut oil and place the balls in a skillet pan and cook for 15 minutes until golden brown.
- Prepare a pot to cook the sauce and set heat to medium high.
- Add olive oil, garlic, pepper, onions, parsley, cayenne and cumin.
- Cook for about 10 minutes, then add the cooked meatballs and simmer for 15 minutes.
- Serve the spicy meatballs with sourdough bread on the side.

DASH DIET RECIPES

Baked chicken and wild rice with onion and tarragona

Ingredients:

1 pound boneless, skinless chicken breasts halves

1 1/2 cups sliced celery

1 1/2 mugs whole pearl onions

1 teaspoon new tarragon

2 mugs saltless chicken broth

1 1/2 glasses free of moisture bright white red wine

3/4 mug uncooked very long grain rice

3/4 mug uncooked crazy rice

DIRECTIONS:

Pre-heat the oven to 300 F.

Minimize chicken breast bosoms into 1/2- to 1-in . pieces. Mix thechicken and celery, pearl onions and tarragon in addition 1 glass of the unsalted chicken broth in the non-stick frying pan. Cook on medium sized heat until the vegetables and chicken are sensitive, about 10-20 minutes. Set aside to great.

Within a cooking meal, merge the wine, remaining 1 mug chicken breast broth, and rice. Permit soak for thirty minutes.

Add more the cooked vegetables and chicken towards the preparing recipe. Deal with and bake for 60 minutes. Check periodically and add more broth if the rice is too dry. Offer right away.

Broccoli, garlic and rigatoni

Ingredients:

1/3 pound rigatoni noodles
2 glasses broccoli florets (tops)
2 tablespoons Parmesan cheese
2 teaspoons olive oil
2 teaspoons minced garlic clove
Recently soil dark pepper, to taste

Directions:

Fill up a huge pot 3/4 whole with water and convey into a boil. Put the pasta and cook right up until al dente (soft), 10 to 12 a few minutes, or in accordance with the bundle recommendations. Drain the noodles extensively.
Whilst the spaghetti is food preparation, in the cooking pot installed having a steamer basket, take 1 inches of water to some boil. Add more the steam, cover and broccoli until tender, about ten minutes.

Within a big container, merge the cooked pasta and broccoli. Toss with Parmesan cheddar cheese, essential olive oil and garlic herb. Period with pepper to style. Provide quickly.